Clinical Practice to Academia

A Guide for New and Aspiring Health Professions Faculty

Clinical Practice to Academia

A Guide for New and Aspiring Health Professions Faculty

Crystal A. Gateley, PhD, OTR/L
Associate Chair
Teaching Professor
Department of Occupational Therapy
University of Missouri
Columbia, Missouri

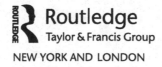

Routledge
Taylor & Francis Group

NEW YORK AND LONDON

Cover Artist: Christine Seabo

Dr. Crystal A. Gateley has no financial or proprietary interest in the materials presented herein.

First published in 2021 by SLACK Incorporated

Published in 2024 by Routledge
605 Third Avenue, New York, NY 10158

and by Routledge
4 Park Square, Milton Park, Abingdon, Oxon, OX14 4RN

Routledge is an imprint of the Taylor & Francis Group, an informa business

© 2021 Taylor & Francis Group

Library of Congress Cataloging-in-Publication Data

Names: Gateley, Crystal A., 1974- author.
Title: Clinical practice to academia : a guide for new and aspiring health
    professions faculty / Crystal A. Gateley.
Description: Thorofare, NJ : SLACK Incorporated, [2021] | Includes
    bibliographical references and index.
Identifiers: LCCN 2020022017 (print) | ISBN 9781630914363 (paperback)

Subjects: MESH: Faculty, Medical | Education, Medical | Professional Role |
    Teaching
Classification: LCC R697.A4 (print) | NLM W 19.1 |
    DDC 610.69--dc23
LC record available at https://lccn.loc.gov/2020022017

ISBN: 9781630914363 (pbk)
ISBN: 9781003523123 (ebk)

DOI: 10.4324/9781003523123

DEDICATION

This book is dedicated to all the health professions students across the country whose educational experiences were impacted by the COVID-19 pandemic. Courses transitioned from in-person, hands-on experiences to online learning overnight. Clinical and fieldwork experiences were cancelled or postponed. Graduations were delayed. Yet you persevered. You did what you needed to do to achieve your dreams of becoming a health care professional. My hope is that in your career, some of you will find a love for teaching like I did, and that you will find this book helpful when you decide to consider a transition to academia.

CONTENTS

ACKNOWLEDGMENTS

I would like to thank Brien Cummings, Senior Acquisitions Editor, who believed in this project from the moment I suggested it way back in 2013 and was persistent in presenting it to the SLACK Incorporated leadership team until it was approved. Thank you for your unwavering patience over the past few years as I have encountered too many life challenges to mention! Thank you also to the entire SLACK Incorporated team for each part you played in bringing this book to fruition.

I am grateful for the support of all my departmental colleagues at University of Missouri: Tim Wolf, Lea Ann Lowery, Rachel Proffitt, Gina Pifer, Stephanie Allen, Anna Boone, Tiffany Bolton, Whitney Henderson, Brittney Stevenson, Bill Janes, Winnie Dunn, Sam Shea Lemoins, Bailey Baucum, Bethany Kendrick, Angie Williams, Lynn Herdzina, Beth Voyles, and Byron Smith. I am blessed to work in a collaborative environment where excellence in occupational therapy practice, education, and research are valued and respected. I am also thankful for my colleagues and friends "down the hall" in the Department of Physical Therapy and across the School of Health Professions. Your friendship and support make it a joy to come to work, even during some of the most challenging times in my personal life. Special thanks to Jamie Hall for following me to three different jobs over the past 20 years, the many lunch dates at Chipotle and Campus Bar & Grill, and all the years of mutual support through graduate school, job transitions, and kid-raising adventures!

I would also like to acknowledge Joe Sadewhite and my dozens of OT, PT, and SLP colleagues at Boone Hospital Center for your friendship, support, and last-minute shift coverage when I needed it over the past few years. I am blessed to have not one but two jobs that I love.

There was a point in early 2019 at which I wondered if this manuscript would ever get completed. Life threw more personal challenges at my family at one time than I thought we could handle. It was during this time that we experienced the true meaning of friendship. When nothing in life seemed normal and others "outside our circle" didn't really know what to say or do, we had a core group of friends who never failed to make us laugh and who would drop everything to lend a hand when needed. Thank you to Myles and Lora Hinkel, Mark and Ustena Simenson, Russ and Jamie Drury, Whitney Payne, James Scurlock, Michael Abbott, Bill and Christy Adams, John and Angela Schultz, and Trent and Sarah Gateley. Thank you to Erick Taylor for the weekly *Survivor* nights and for always listening to and supporting me through life's ups and downs. Last but not least, huge thank you to my friend of nearly 30 years, Michelle Bass, who always knows exactly the right moment to demand a 2-hour hike or to show up unexpectedly with my favorite frozen beverage. With the support of these many friends, I was able to regain my writing mojo and find my "new normal" long before it became one of the most overused phrases of 2020.

A big thank you goes out to the many University of Missouri occupational therapy students who have helped me learn how to be a better teacher, beginning with the graduating Class of 2009 up through my current cohorts. A special thank you to the Classes of 2019 and 2020 who were so supportive to me personally and patient with the many changes to their courses while I was balancing teaching with life's many curveballs. I am honored to consider you both colleagues and friends.

I want to acknowledge my parents, Dave and Eileen Aldridge, whose lives were also turned upside down over the last few years. Through the many trials and tribulations of selling our respective homes, buying a house together, and combining households, your love and support have been unconditional. I am glad we are finally all under one roof!

Most importantly, I would like to thank my husband, Curt, and my two daughters, Katrina and Lauren, for your continued patience, love, and support through all of my educational and professional endeavors. Curt, thank you for the most wonderful 25 years of marriage and for making me laugh every day. I love you so much! Katrina, while working on this book, I have watched you achieve so many things at University of Mississippi, and I'm sorry that your 2020 graduation didn't turn out as expected. I can't wait to see where you end up for graduate school for the next few years and what you accomplish next. Lauren, I am so happy that your dream of attending University of Tennessee came true in 2018, all through your own hard work and dedication. You missed out on so many college plans in 2020, but I hope that your last 2 years of undergrad are everything you hoped for. I am excited to see what life will bring next for you. Words cannot describe how proud I am of both of you!

ABOUT THE AUTHOR

Crystal A. Gateley, PhD, OTR/L is Associate Chair and Teaching Professor at the University of Missouri, Department of Occupational Therapy, where she has taught full-time since 2009. She teaches a variety of courses across the curriculum including Foundations and Theory in Occupational Therapy, Conditions in Occupational Therapy, Psychosocial Aspects of Occupational Therapy, Clinical Reasoning and Documentation, Emerging Trends in Occupational Therapy, and Leadership, Management, and Policy. She also has taught interdisciplinary courses including Clinical Pathophysiology and Introduction to the Health Professions. In her administrative role, she provides oversight of curriculum revision and accreditation compliance, and she assists with new program development and the myriad of issues faced by a growing department.

Crystal graduated Summa Cum Laude from the University of Missouri in 1995 with a BHS in Occupational Therapy. She went on to complete a master's (2003) and doctorate (2015) in Educational Leadership and Policy Analysis, also from the University of Missouri. Crystal has worked in a variety of occupational therapy practice settings, including acute care, inpatient and outpatient rehabilitation, skilled nursing, home health, outpatient pediatrics, public schools, and community programs for adults with developmental disabilities. She still provides occasional occupational therapy coverage at Boone Hospital Center in Columbia, Missouri, on weekends and holidays, and her experiences there with patients and interprofessional colleagues inform her teaching as she is able to pass along insights from contemporary occupational therapy practice to her students.

Beyond her love for college teaching and occupational therapy practice, Crystal enjoys spending time with friends and family in outdoor activities including camping, fishing, canoeing, and rafting along various Missouri rivers. She is an avid football fan, and she is still basking in the glory of the Kansas City Chiefs' Super Bowl LIV victory in 2020! She currently lives in rural Holts Summit, Missouri, with her husband, Curt, and her parents. Crystal treasures the occasional phone calls and visits from her two daughters, Katrina and Lauren, who are off on their own college adventures.

1

Introduction

As you prepare to read this book, I think it is helpful first to know a little bit about my approach to writing. My writing style has been described as "informal" and "conversational," and I have received good feedback from students and colleagues on past writing endeavors. "It was like you were talking to me. That made it so easy to read and understand," a student once said to me about a previous textbook I coauthored. In my opinion, that is the best compliment an author could ever hope to receive. "Easy to read and understand"—shouldn't that be the goal of writing a textbook? Some academics may find my informality a bit off putting, but I am not writing this for them. I am writing it for you. You have purchased or somehow acquired this textbook, so my guess is that you fall into one of the three following categories of potential readers:

1. You are a health care professional hoping to transition into an academic role in the future, and you are looking for helpful advice about how to make that transition.
2. You are a health care professional who recently has transitioned into an academic role, and after a few months or years of feeling like you have little to no idea what you are doing, you are seeking out resources and stumbled across this book.
3. You are a graduate student enrolled in a course, or perhaps an entire degree program, dedicated to learning how to be an educator in the health professions.

I may have missed a few readers with these categories, but those were the groups I had in mind when I first decided to write this book. Whatever your situation, I hope that you find the contents of this book useful in some way.

Gateley, C. A. *Clinical Practice to Academia:*
A Guide for New and Aspiring Health Professions Faculty
(pp. 1-7). © 2021 Taylor & Francis Group.

College teaching is a lot like first-time parenting. Many people have done it successfully before you, but just as many have messed up royally. I think most parents want to do a good job, and those who have the right mix of determination, support, resilience, and resources do just fine. I think the same is true for college educators. You must have the desire to be a good teacher and the resilience to keep trying to improve even when things do not turn out as well as you had hoped. As for support and resources, those factors will vary greatly depending on your setting. They do exist, but you often have to seek them out for yourself.

This book is intended to serve as a resource for health care professionals transitioning from clinical practice to an academic role. It is a synthesis of lessons I have learned throughout my own professional journey—lessons that I hope will be helpful to others as they encounter similar challenges. I draw upon several of the resources I have found over the years through graduate education, professional development programs, and literature on contemporary health care and education. As you read this book, if you think of other resources that should be included in the next edition, please let me know! You should be able to find my current work e-mail through a simple online search, or you can send me a message through SLACK Incorporated.

AUTHOR'S BACKGROUND

I completed an undergraduate degree in occupational therapy in 1995. Back then, a bachelor's degree was all that was required to practice as an occupational therapist. I will discuss the concept of *degree creep* more in Chapter 2. I worked for 14 years in a variety of practice settings including inpatient acute and rehabilitation hospitals, outpatient pediatric clinics, skilled nursing facilities, home health, early intervention, and school-based practice. In addition to the joy that I got from helping my clients achieve their goals, another favorite aspect of my professional role was serving as a fieldwork educator to students who were enrolled in occupational therapy educational programs. I discovered that I loved teaching!

I stayed in close contact with my alma mater, providing guest lectures, helping with labs, and even teaching an entire course on an adjunct basis. I sought the advice of former professors about how to pursue a full-time academic role in the future. Their collective message was simple—more education. It did not matter how much experience I had as an occupational therapist; without at least a master's degree, I would have no chance of landing a job in an occupational therapy education program. Unbeknownst to me at the time, my profession was already undergoing changes at the national level—changes that would dictate the need for advanced degrees for both clinical practitioners and educators.

I completed a master's degree in Educational Leadership and Policy Analysis in 2003. At that point, I had only 8 years of clinical experience. I did not yet feel qualified to go teach the next generation of occupational therapists, so I remained in clinical practice for several more years. I finally made the leap into a full-time academic position in 2009. By then, I had mentored dozens of students in various settings, and I thought I had a pretty good idea of what I was getting myself into. Turns out I was very naive.

Can you imagine sending a child to an elementary, middle, or high school filled with teachers who had never received any formal training in teaching? Ridiculous, right? Yet that's the reality of many college educators. They are content experts, but no one ever taught them how to teach. Yes, I may have been considered a seasoned expert in clinical practice and even a great fieldwork educator, but I quickly discovered that I had no idea what I was doing in the classroom. I wanted to be a good educator. I had students and their parents paying for my courses. I felt obligated to them, their future clients, and my profession to be a good educator, but I didn't know how to find the help I needed. Honestly, I didn't even know what help I was looking for, much less how to find it!

Don't get me wrong, I worked at a great institution with very supportive colleagues, but at the time there were no formal mentorship or orientation programs for new teaching faculty. There was a 2-day campus-wide orientation for new faculty during my first week, but that program focused mostly on tenure-track faculty (more on that in Chapter 3), and I did not even get to attend that orientation because my department had a faculty retreat scheduled at the exact same time. After a few semesters of feeling like I was floundering in my new academic role and reading my less than stellar course evaluations, I knew I had to do something.

In clinical practice, when you encounter a new diagnosis, practice setting, billing policy, or anything unfamiliar, what do you do? You educate yourself, right? Surely there must be a book, a website, an academic journal, a continuing education conference, a specialty certification, or a mentor whose brain you can pick for answers, so that's what I did. I started searching for answers, but they did not come neatly bundled in a single article, website, book, course, conference, or mentor. I had to work hard to find them, and I had to piece them together a little at a time. I attended continuing education conferences related to college teaching. I read books and articles about college teaching. I applied for every professional development opportunity my campus had to offer for early career faculty. I completed a PhD in Educational Leadership and Policy Analysis, incorporating several courses and self-directed learning experiences on instructional design, understanding college students, and understanding the professoriate. I focused my dissertation research on understanding the professional development needs of early career faculty. What I discovered along the way is that my situation as a struggling academic was not unique or unusual. Rather, it was the norm for many new faculty.

In retrospect, I realize that I was approaching my transition from clinician to academician from the wrong perspective. Just like new parents do not cease identifying with all the previous life roles they held before parenthood, the transition from clinical practice to academia is not really a change from one specific role to another (Figure 1-1). It is more like a gradual blending of old and new roles, resulting in an expanded identity. Just as new personal life roles become a part of your overall identity so do new professional roles (Figure 1-2). New roles may become a more central part of your identity or take up more time and effort than your previous roles, but many of those other roles will still remain if they are important to you. Taking this line of reasoning one step further, you likely have already discovered that it is impossible to completely separate personal and professional roles. Each role simply

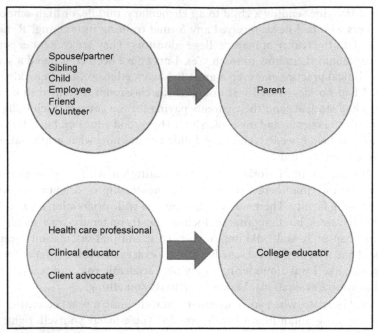

Figure 1-1. An unrealistic view of transitioning to new personal or professional roles.

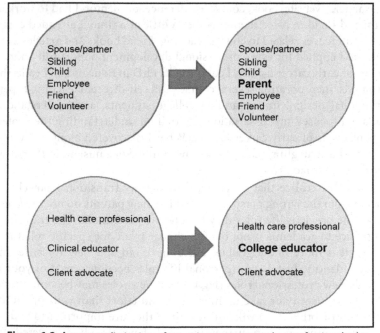

Figure 1-2. A more realistic view of assuming new personal or professional roles.

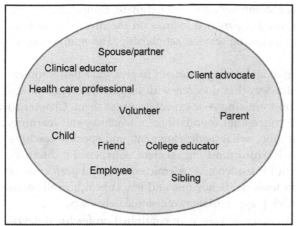

Figure 1-3. An overlap and integration of personal and professional roles into overall identity.

becomes a part of your larger overall identity (Figure 1-3). In no way am I implying that the personal and professional roles listed in these figures are the only or most important roles that you may have. Each individual reading this book could create a unique graphic representation of his or her specific combination of roles. The roles listed were selected simply for illustrative purposes.

ORGANIZATION OF BOOK

Chapter 2 provides a brief overview of the health care context in which we, as educators, are preparing students to practice. Drawing from professional experience and national resources on public health promotion, I discuss several issues affecting practitioners and educators. Chapter 3 reviews contemporary issues specific to higher education, including funding, globalization, technology, and interprofessional education. I also discuss legal issues in higher education, various faculty types, faculty salaries, and issues related to women and minority faculty.

Chapter 4 introduces various institutional types as defined by The Carnegie Classification of Institutions of Higher Education. The intent of this brief chapter is to provide readers with the resources to explore more information about institutions of interest to them. Chapter 5 covers key issues related to pursuing an academic job, including how to locate faculty positions, the application and interview process, and how to negotiate salary and benefits.

Chapter 6 provides guidance about knowing your profession beyond any clinical experience you may have. To be an effective health professions educator, you need to be familiar with relevant professional associations, accreditation standards, certification and licensure requirements, professional publications, and the guiding documents of your profession. Chapter 7 gives you numerous suggestions about becoming familiar with your campus, school, and department throughout your first year in an academic position. I include brief discussions about institutional governance, organizational theory, campus culture and climate, campus resources, and promotion and tenure guidelines. Chapter 8 focuses on the diverse aspects of the faculty role beyond teaching, including service, scholarship, and many student-related responsibilities.

Chapter 9 reviews literature on today's college students to give you a better understanding of why students behave the way they do along with suggestions about how to teach them effectively without compromising your expectations for them. Chapter 10 provides a brief overview of the conceptual foundations of teaching and learning. Chapter 11 covers course preparation, syllabus development, and specific teaching approaches to facilitate student learning and engagement. Chapter 12 discusses professional behavior development for students. Academic and clinical performance can be overshadowed by poor professional behaviors, and we, as health professions educators, must help students develop appropriate professional behaviors.

Chapter 13 returns the focus to you and your own continued professional development. Just as health care practitioners should continue learning new strategies throughout their years in clinical practice, college educators should always be looking for ways to expand their knowledge and skills as educators and scholars. Chapter 14 takes a look at the important concept of maintaining balance in your life. In other words, how do you successfully balance your academic position with the many other roles in your life?

Although my experience as both a clinician and an educator is in the occupational therapy profession, I believe the topics covered in this book are relevant across health professions education. You may be an expert in your field, but you may have received little guidance or experience about college teaching. This book is certainly not the only resource that you need to become an effective faculty member. Rather, I intend it to be a starting point for you. In each chapter, I provide several suggestions of learning activities that will encourage you to explore resources specific to your profession or institution. If you are a student in a graduate course, your instructor may assign some of these activities to you and your classmates. If you are not a student and have instead sought out this resource on your own, I challenge you to complete at least a few of the learning activities that seem most relevant to your unique situation. If you read this entire book in order, you may notice some occasional redundancy between chapters. I wrote this book with the expectation that some individuals will read the entire book, whereas others may read only select chapters that are most relevant to them.

LEARNING ACTIVITIES

1. Create a list or graphic representation of your current personal and professional roles. How will those roles change, or how have they changed, with a transition to academia? Which roles will be sacrificed or receive less of your time and energy?
2. Write a letter to someone important in your life. Perhaps a parent, spouse/partner, child, or friend who may receive less of your attention as you embark on this new educational and/or professional journey. Change is never easy, but having an open discussion about what to expect may help reduce the stress on your personal relationships.

3. Write a letter to your future self. At some point in your educational or professional journey, you have likely been asked, "Where do you see yourself in 5 years?" You pick the appropriate time frame. Think about your current goals. Why are you reading this book? Is it because you want to or because a professor said you are required to read it for a course? What do you hope to learn about becoming a health professions educator? What kind of educator do you want to be? Put the letter somewhere safe where you will be able to locate it later. Make a plan to open it and read it in a few years. I have used a similar activity with my occupational therapy students. There are usually a few tears shed when they reread that letter.

4. Think about the best and worst teachers you have had in your life, spanning from preschool to college. Make a list of things that you liked or did not like about their approaches to teaching. Reflect on how these lists will impact how you approach your own role as an educator. If there is a particularly memorable educator who had a positive impact on you, consider sending a note of gratitude to that individual or his or her family if the individual is deceased. There are few things more rewarding for an educator than hearing that he or she changed a student's life or career for the better.

2

The Health Care Context

Although this is one of the first chapters of this book, it was the last one I tackled when writing the manuscript, partly because health care is constantly changing and I wanted you to have the most current information and partly because the idea of trying to summarize the health care context in one concise chapter was a daunting task. As I mentioned in Chapter 1, I assume that most people reading this book have some background knowledge about health care from studying about and working in their respective professions. Whether you are a student or an experienced practitioner, you know the primary issues that affect your profession. This chapter provides a brief overview of some of the most salient topics affecting health care practitioners and educators. The topics that I selected from this chapter come from three primary sources:

- The Healthy People website: The U.S. Department of Health and Human Services (DHHS) Office of Disease Prevention and Health Promotion (ODPHP) maintains the www.healthypeople.gov website, which "provides science-based, 10-year national objectives for improving the health of all Americans" (U.S. DHHS ODPHP, 2019a, para. 1). At the time of this writing, we are nearing the end of the *Healthy People 2020* framework. By the time most of you read this book, *Healthy People 2030* will have been published. I encourage you to take a look at the website to see which topics, goals, and objectives were selected for the new framework. Typically, some topics carry over from decade to decade, whereas new topics will also emerge as the nation's health issues change over time.
- The American Public Health Association (APHA) website (www.apha.org), much like the Healthy People website, strives "to improve access to care, bring about health equity and support public health infrastructure.... We focus on the most important problems and solutions of our time" (APHA, 2018d, para. 1).

Gateley, C. A. *Clinical Practice to Academia: A Guide for New and Aspiring Health Professions Faculty* (pp. 9-21). © 2021 Taylor & Francis Group.

Not surprisingly, there is considerable overlap between the topics published on the U.S. DHHS and APHA websites.

- Professional experience: Between the two websites mentioned, there are dozens of topics and issues relevant to health care practitioners and the general public. It is beyond the scope of this book to provide an in-depth discussion of each topic. Rather, I have selected several topics that have been at the forefront of my recent experience as both a health care practitioner and health professions faculty member. Did I leave out some important topics? Undoubtedly. Would another author have selected an entirely different set of topics? I imagine some topics would be the same no matter who wrote this chapter. My goal here is to provide enough of an overview that you start to see connections between these issues, your profession, and your future role as a faculty member preparing the next generation of health care practitioners.

AGING POPULATION AND CHRONIC CONDITIONS

Americans are living longer, and "growth in the number of older adults is unprecedented. In 2014, 14.5% (46.3 million) of the US population was aged 65 or older and is projected to reach 23.5% (98 million) by 2060" (U.S. DHHS ODPHP, 2019g, para. 1). As the older adult population continues to grow, so do their health needs related to chronic conditions, such as heart disease, cancer, lung disease, stroke, diabetes, and Alzheimer's disease. These conditions may lead to lower quality of life and eventually death. The effects of chronic conditions place considerable strain on caregivers and the health care system.

MATERNAL AND CHILD HEALTH

With advancements in knowledge, science, and technology, health care practitioners have the ability to provide unprecedented levels of care to women, infants, children, and adolescents (APHA, 2018b). Parents can watch their child grow from the first positive pregnancy test to birth through remarkable three- and four-dimensional imaging. Doctors can detect and surgically repair some birth defects in utero to improve the chances of survival and function. Extremely premature babies, who may not have survived a few decades ago, grow up to lead happy, healthy lives.

Despite these many advancements, many women and children have limited or no access to quality health services and health education (APHA, 2018b). Disparities in health care access and outcomes continue to exist among women and children from minority backgrounds and low socioeconomic status. Childhood obesity is on the rise. Adolescents are experiencing mental health issues at alarming rates. These are just a few of the many issues we see in health care settings serving women and children.

COMMUNICABLE DISEASE

As health care providers, regardless of discipline, we should all be concerned about preventing and controlling the spread of disease. Public health efforts include educating people about proper handwashing, avoiding people who are sick, practicing safe sex, ensuring that food and drink are safe for consumption, and getting recommended vaccinations (APHA, 2018a). Yet, we continue to see high numbers of health care–associated infections, spirited political and religious debates over sex education, frequent news stories about food contamination and foodborne illnesses, and growing numbers of Americans refusing immunizations for their children, in large part due to a 1998 study linking autism to childhood vaccines, a study that has long since been retracted after evidence that the lead author falsified data (Rao & Andrade, 2011). As health care practitioners attempt to convince parents to protect their children against diseases once considered eradicated in the United States, they also face new challenges each year with diseases, such as the Zika and Ebola viruses (APHA, 2018a).

I wrote the previous paragraph several months before the onset of the COVID-19 pandemic. I had no idea that a small section in this chapter would turn out to be one of the most pressing issues for both health care and higher education throughout 2020 and the foreseeable future. As I write these words in mid-June 2020, we are just over 3 months into a health care crisis like none of us has seen in our lifetime. Every day brings new stories of how COVID-19 has changed health care. Many hospitals were overwhelmed with patients in critical condition and faced projected or realized shortages of space, staff, and necessary supplies to deal with the influx of patients (Ornstein, 2020). Elective surgeries and other procedures were cancelled or postponed. Outpatient visits were cancelled, postponed, or moved to virtual visits with health care providers. With reduced procedures and visits came reduced revenue, which subsequently resulted in many health care professionals facing layoffs, furlough, salary cuts, or job elimination. Hospitals and residential nursing facilities eliminated or significantly reduced visitors to mitigate risk of bringing the virus into those facilities. Many facilities implemented screening procedures for employees, patients, visitors, vendors, and anyone else who enters the building. With no end in sight to this pandemic at the time of this writing, COVID-19 is certain to be remembered as one of the most historical health care events of this century, and it will be interesting to see the long lasting changes in our health care system once an effective vaccine and/or treatment is found.

SUBSTANCE MISUSE

Substance misuse "includes the use of illegal drugs and the inappropriate use of legal substances, such as alcohol and tobacco" (APHA, 2018c, para. 1). The misuse of and addiction to opioids has risen to a national crisis according to the National Institute on Drug Abuse (2019). Every day hundreds of people are hospitalized or die from overdosing on prescription pain relievers, heroin, and fentanyl, resulting in an economic burden of nearly $80 billion dollars per year for the costs of health care, lost productivity, and involvement in the criminal justice system. In nearly any health care setting, you are likely to encounter someone who is dealing with substance misuse and addiction.

INJURY AND VIOLENCE PREVENTION

In the United States, unintentional injuries and acts of violence are among the top 10 causes of death for all age groups (APHA, 2013). Falls are a leading cause of injury and death in older adults. Motor vehicle accidents affect all age groups, and smartphone technology has led to increased concerns for distracted driving (U.S. DHHS ODPHP, 2019e). Homicide related to gang violence, domestic abuse, substance misuse, and other circumstances is a leading cause of death among those 15 to 24 years of age, with significant disparities among those from minority populations and low socioeconomic status (APHA, 2013). "But injuries are not only killing us, they are sending us to hospitals and emergency rooms for critical care and to social service agencies to file disability claims" (APHA, 2013, p. 2). Individuals who have experienced injury or violence have complex health and psychosocial needs that health professions students need to be prepared to address when they enter their professions.

LESBIAN, GAY, BISEXUAL, AND TRANSGENDER HEALTH

Individuals who are members of the lesbian, gay, bisexual, transgender, and queer (LGBTQ) community often face "health disparities linked to societal stigma, discrimination, and denial of their civil and human rights" (U.S. DHHS ODPHP, 2019f, para. 3). LGBTQ individuals experience violence, victimization, and lack of acceptance by family and society for their gender identity or sexual orientation, leading to increased mental health issues and reluctance to seek health care. They may also experience legal discrimination in access to employment, health insurance, and retirement benefits resulting in decreased economic stability, which in turn is linked to poorer health outcomes. Students entering health professions need to learn how to address the health care needs of the LGBTQ population with competence and compassion. Faculty teaching in health professions programs may have limited knowledge and experience themselves working with LGBTQ individuals and will need to seek out other campus and community resources to address student learning needs with this population.

GLOBAL HEALTH

Most of your future students will practice their professions in the United States, although a few may already have aspirations to complete international clinicals, fieldwork, or health care mission trips or seek out employment in another country. Regardless of their eventual practice settings, all future health care practitioners need to understand global health issues (U.S. DHHS ODPHP, 2019c). Infectious diseases and foodborne illnesses spread easily through international travel and trade. Bioterrorism is a growing threat to global security. There are worldwide disparities in access to adequate food supplies, clean drinking water, and health care services for the prevention and treatment of noncommunicable and infectious diseases. Furthermore, individuals from various cultural and religious backgrounds may have different knowledge, beliefs, and expectations about health care that impact how practitioners provide care to them.

SOCIAL DETERMINANTS OF HEALTH

"The conditions in which you live, learn, work and age affect your health. Social determinants such as neighborhood, education and health care can influence your lifelong well-being" (APHA, 2019, para. 1). The conditions in which we live help explain why some Americans are generally in better health than others (U.S. DHHS ODPHP, 2019h). Examples of social determinants include the availability of food and housing, access to education and employment, availability of community recreation resources, transportation options, social supports, socioeconomic conditions, culture, social norms and attitudes, incidence of crime and violence, residential segregation, language and literacy, and access to technology.

> Since social determinants, such as race, income, and environment strongly influence who becomes ill and who receives access to quality health care, the health care crisis disproportionately affects disadvantaged groups and under-resourced communities, such as people living in poverty, people of color, and immigrants. (National Economic & Social Rights Initiative, 2018, para. 2)

Health outcomes are also affected by health literacy or "the degree to which individuals have the capacity to obtain, process, and understand basic health information and services needed to make appropriate health decisions" (U.S. DHHS ODPHP, n.d., p. 4). Students in health professions programs need to understand the many global health issues that affect their roles as future health practitioners.

ACCESS TO HEALTH SERVICES

Closely linked to social determinants of health is whether or not an individual has access to comprehensive, quality health services, including oral health care and the ability to obtain necessary prescription medications (U.S. DHHS ODPHP, 2019b). Access to health services involves the following three components:

1. Insurance coverage or other funding to access the health care system
2. Availability of health care services within a geographically accessible area
3. Finding a health care provider who the individual trusts in a timely manner to address health care needs

Access to health services is one of the issues that has been at the forefront of U.S. politics for decades. The Patient Protection and Affordable Care Act of 2010 helped provide health insurance coverage to an additional 20 million Americans. Yet, millions of others remain uninsured or underinsured, and health care access remains a contentious issue for legislators, political candidates, and the general public. Health professions students and educators must stay abreast of recent and proposed legislation that impacts access to health care for individuals needing the services of their respective professions.

TECHNOLOGY IN HEALTH CARE

Technology affects health care services and health outcomes in countless ways. "Health communication and health information technology (IT) are central to health care, public health, and the way our society views health" (U.S. DHHS ODPHP, 2019d, para. 2). Professionals and the general public use technology to locate, understand, and use health information. A new mother may perform an online search of her baby's symptoms or chat online with a nurse to determine if she should take the baby to the emergency department. A physician may pull up the results of a computed tomographic scan or magnetic resonance imaging to explain to a patient and family where in the brain a stroke occurred and how it will affect the patient's function. A respiratory therapist will rely on physician orders placed in a patient's electronic health record to guide the frequency and dosage for a patient's breathing treatments. A physical therapist assistant may perform real-time documentation on a tablet or laptop as a patient performs guided postsurgical exercises in an outpatient clinic. A patient may log in to his or her own electronic health record to access notes from clinic visits or to send a question via email to his or her health care provider. A health professions educator may rely on computerized simulation equipment to give students the opportunity to develop and practice skills before working with clients. The list of possibilities goes on and on. As a health professions educator, you will need to stay informed about the latest technological advances in your field in order to prepare your students for entry-level practice.

EVIDENCE-BASED PRACTICE

As a health professions student or practitioner, you certainly have heard the term *evidence-based practice*. If asked to define evidence-based practice, most of us would say something to the effect of making sure that our practice decisions are based on the most current research. However, evidence-based practice also involves a practitioner's clinical expertise, information from the practice context, and the patient's values and circumstances.

> Evidence-based practice is not just about using research evidence.... It is also about valuing and using the education, skills and experience that you have as a health professional. Furthermore, and just as importantly, it is also about considering the patient's situation and values when making a decision, as well as considering the characteristics of the practice context (for example, the resources available). This requires judgment and artistry, as well as science and logic. The process that health professionals use to integrate all of this information is clinical reasoning.... When you take these four elements and combine them in a way that enables you to make decisions about the care of a patient, then you are engaging in evidence-based practice. (Hoffman, Bennett, & Del Mar, 2017, pp. 3-4)

DEGREE CREEP

Another issue permeating health care is *degree creep*, also known as *credential creep*, *credentialism*, and *educational inflation*. "Degree creep refers to mandating that a higher degree now be attained to perform the same job that formerly required a lower degree" (Kibe & Cawley, 2018, p. 403). For example, when I graduated in 1995, a bachelor's degree was the entry-level degree required to practice as an occupational therapist. By 2007, a master's degree was the mandated entry-level degree for occupational therapists. Now my profession is in the midst of a debate about whether a clinical doctorate should be the mandated entry-level degree for occupational therapists, and many educational programs have already made the transition (American Occupational Therapy Association, 2018). Other health professions have seen similar increases in the degree for entry-level practice. Clinical doctorates are now required for entry-level nurse practitioners, physical therapists, and pharmacists, and they are under consideration for physician assistants (Kibe & Cawley, 2018). Other health professions are also transitioning or considering transitioning from requiring a bachelor's degree to a master's degree or from requiring a technical or associate's degree to requiring a bachelor's degree.

Why the push for higher degrees to do the same job previously performed by individuals with less education? Requiring a higher-level degree, and therefore a longer period of time in school, allows students more time to develop clinical competence and confidence as they prepare to enter complex health care environments (Kibe & Cawley, 2018; Palmer, Doig, & Konkin, 2017). Advanced degrees also provide students with increased training in research and leadership skills, thus allowing them the opportunity for expanded career roles beyond clinical practice. As other professions make the transition to advanced degrees, professions that require lower-level degrees risk being less respected and perhaps reimbursed at lower levels for the services they provide.

Although there are many benefits to health professions requiring advanced education, degree creep also comes with many challenges, including longer time to degree completion, lack of uniformity among educational programs in terms of degree requirements, increased student debt without a guaranteed salary increase, workforce shortages, lack of qualified faculty, and risk of widening the diversity gap across health care professions (Kibe & Cawley, 2018). "The high cost/slow yield for some health care educations might also make great, would-be practitioners reconsider entering certain fields altogether" (Garvin, 2012, para. 9). There is also a growing concern that community colleges will no longer be able to offer students affordable access to health professions careers because associate's degrees are being devalued (Fulcher, 2009).

Transition to higher entry-level degree requirements often involves controversy and confusion for students, educators, practitioners, employers, and the general public. When my profession moved to an entry-level master's degree, I had over a decade of experience with my bachelor's degree, but suddenly I had fieldwork students who questioned if I was qualified to supervise them because they were getting a master's degree. The same students were later upset to learn that they would not be receiving a higher salary as an entry-level occupational therapist even though they spent more time and money to earn their degrees. Whether or not overtly discussed, there may be a wariness among colleagues with different level degrees. "Does she think she's better than me just because she has different letters behind her name?" "Does he really engage in evidence-based practice because he didn't receive the research training that I did?"

These issues also affect the educational programs that prepare students for practice. As entry-level degree requirements increase, so do the requirements for faculty and educational administrators. It may not matter that you have 20 years of clinical experience and 10 years of experience as a faculty member. You still may need to obtain a postprofessional degree in order to meet the educational accreditation requirements for your profession.

Shortages in Health Professions Practitioners and Faculty

The U.S. Department of Labor's Bureau of Labor Statistics (2019) maintains an online *Occupational Outlook Handbook*, which provides information about various careers, including entry-level degree requirements, median salary, and future job outlook. Table 2-1 shows that most health professions were predicted to experience growth either faster than average or much faster than average between 2016 and 2026, suggesting a steady supply of jobs for students entering the health professions.

TABLE 2-1

PROJECTED GROWTH OF JOBS IN HEALTH PROFESSIONS

HEALTH PROFESSION	PROJECTED EMPLOYMENT GROWTH 2016–2026 (%)	COMPARISON OF EMPLOYMENT GROWTH TO AVERAGE FOR ALL CAREERS
Athletic trainers	23	Much faster than average
Audiologists	21	Much faster than average
Chiropractors	12	Faster than average
Dental hygienists	20	Much faster than average
Dentists	19	Much faster than average
Diagnostic medical sonographers and cardiovascular technologists	17	Much faster than average
Dietitians and nutritionists	15	Much faster than average
Licensed practical nurses	12	Faster than average
Medical laboratory scientists	13	Faster than average
Nuclear medicine technologists	10	Faster than average
Nurse anesthetists, nurse midwives, and nurse practitioners	31	Much faster than average
Occupational therapists	24	Much faster than average
Occupational therapy assistants	28	Much faster than average
Optometrists	18	Much faster than average
Orthotists and prosthetists	22	Much faster than average
Pharmacists	6	As fast as average
Physical therapists	28	Much faster than average
Physical therapist assistants	30	Much faster than average
Physicians and surgeons	13	Faster than average
Physician assistants	37	Much faster than average
Radiation therapists	13	Faster than average
Radiologic and MRI technologists	13	Faster than average
Recreational therapists	7	As fast as average
Registered nurses	15	Much faster than average
Respiratory therapists	23	Much faster than average
Speech-language pathologists	18	Much faster than average
Surgical technologists	12	Faster than average

MRI = magnetic resonance imaging.

Adapted from U.S. Department of Labor's Bureau of Labor Statistics. (2019). *Occupational outlook handbook*. Retrieved from https://www.bls.gov/ooh

Unfortunately, this means that most health professions will continue to experience shortages in qualified practitioners to meet the demand for health care services.

In response to the growing demand for health professionals across all disciplines, new health professions education programs are opening in institutions across the nation, and many existing programs are expanding their enrollment (University of California, 2013). This rapid expansion in health professions education programs in turn leads to a lack of qualified faculty to teach students in those programs. A recent survey of the CEOs of nationwide academic health centers "found that 94% of CEOs think faculty shortages are a problem in at least one health professions school, and 69 percent think that these shortages are a problem for the entire institution" (Association of Academic Health Centers, 2019, para. 1). In addition to health professions program expansion, other factors leading to faculty shortages include retirement of baby boomer faculty, a lack of interest in academic careers, and the fact that many health professionals can make more money in clinical practice than in higher education. For you, as a new or aspiring faculty member, this means you likely will experience greater job security than college educators in many other disciplines outside the health professions. However, the Association of Academic Health Centers paints a more dire picture of what faculty shortages mean for the overall health care environment, suggesting that "a crisis looms: without enough faculty members to teach the next generation of health professionals, the nation's health infrastructure is in jeopardy" (2019, para. 2).

LEARNING ACTIVITIES

1. Explore the Healthy People (www.healthpeople.gov) and American Public Health Association (www.apha.org) websites. Which topics addressed on these websites are most relevant for your profession? Why?
2. Identify health care–related issues that are hot topics in politics and the news right now.
   a. How might these issues affect your profession or those individuals your profession serves?
   b. Explore health care and insurance legislation currently up for consideration at state and national levels. Does your profession have a vested interest in any of this legislation? Is your state or national professional association involved in any advocacy efforts related to legislation?
3. Reflect on your own health care needs and health insurance situation. Compare with others.
   a. What health care or insurance issues do you and your family face? Has someone in your family had an illness or injury lately? Does someone you love have a chronic condition or disability? Do you have access to health care? How much do you spend each year on insurance premiums, deductibles, copays, and other health care expenses? What do you find most frustrating about our health care system as a patient? As a provider?
   b. Talk to some older adults or individuals with a disability or chronic health issues. Ask them these same questions. How do their responses differ from yours?

4. Explore health care services that are available in your area for individuals with limited financial and insurance resources?
   a. Are any of them relevant to your particular discipline?
   b. What is the funding mechanism for these services?
   c. How do people qualify for and access services?
5. Research websites and publications specific to your discipline.
   a. What are some salient issues for your profession?
   b. Can you find anything related to evidence-based practice for your profession? Does your profession have a specific definition or guidelines for evidence-based practice?
   c. Does your profession publish a workforce survey or similar document that describes employment trends and salaries?
6. Search the U.S. Department of Labor's Bureau of Labor Statistics *Occupational Outlook Handbook* online at www.bls.gov/ooh
   a. What is the median pay for your profession? Are you surprised by this?
   b. What is the job outlook for your profession? How does it compare with the job outlook for other health professions?
7. What are some recent and emerging trends for your profession? This discussion will be enhanced if you have a group of individuals with various levels of experience in a particular health profession. A practitioner with 20 years of experience who is just returning to higher education will have very different responses than an individual who has been in a health professions education program more recently.
8. Explore health outcomes for your state.
   a. How do they compare with the rest of the nation?
   b. How can your profession impact those health outcomes?
9. Explore whether degree creep is an issue for your profession. Has the entry-level degree for your profession changed in recent years? Is there discussion within your profession about future changes to entry-level degrees?
10. Explore issues related to practitioner and faculty shortages in your profession.
    a. Are there practitioner shortages in your profession? Are those shortages more prevalent in particular practice areas or geographic locations?
    b. What is the outlook for faculty jobs in your profession? Are there concerns for shortages? What is your profession doing to attract and train individuals for faculty and administrator positions?
11. Explore how the COVID-19 pandemic affected your health profession. Talk with leaders in practice settings to find out about how and why decisions were made. Read recent news articles on your state and national professional associations' websites. Look for blogs, social media groups, or publications relevant to your profession. Discuss what you found with someone from another profession to compare similarities and differences.

REFERENCES

American Occupational Therapy Association. (2018). *ACOTE 2027 mandate update and time-line*. Retrieved from https://www.aota.org/Education-Careers/Accreditation/acote-doctoral-mandate-2027.aspx

American Public Health Association. (2013). *Injury and violence prevention: Policy lessons from the field*. Retrieved from https://www.apha.org/-/media/files/pdf/topics/injury_and_violence_prevention_policy_lessons_from_the_field.ashx?la=en&hash=5FDC317A1C2138662C81E6B19C46C7E029CB3FB1

American Public Health Association. (2018a). *Communicable disease*. Retrieved from https://www.apha.org/topics-and-issues/communicable-disease

American Public Health Association. (2018b). *Maternal and child health*. Retrieved from https://www.apha.org/topics-and-issues/maternal-and-child-health

American Public Health Association. (2018c). *Substance misuse*. Retrieved from https://www.apha.org/topics-and-issues/substance-misuse

American Public Health Association. (2018d). *Topics and issues*. Retrieved from https://www.apha.org/topics-and-issues

American Public Health Association. (2019). *Social determinants of health*. Retrieved from http://thenationshealth.aphapublications.org/content/nations-health-series-social-determinants-health

Association of Academic Health Centers. (2019). *Academic health center CEOs say faculty shortages threaten health workforce*. Retrieved from https://www.aahcdc.org/Publications-Resources/Series/Issue-Briefs/View/ArticleId/15970/Academic-Health-Center-CEOs-Say-Faculty-Shortages-Threaten-Health-Workforce

Fulcher, R. (2009). Fighting degree creep: AACC fights to protect access to the health professions at community colleges. *Community College Journal, 79*(4), 28-30.

Garvin, K. (2012, November 14). "Degree creep" and the cost of health care education. *Huffington Post*. Retrieved from https://www.huffingtonpost.com/kathleen-garvin/degree-creep-and-the-cost_b_2130347.html

Hoffman, T., Bennett, T., & Del Mar, C. (2017). Introduction to evidence-based practice. In T. Hoffman, S. Bennett, & C. Del Mar (Eds.), *Evidence-based practice across the health professions* (3rd ed., pp. 1-15). New South Wales, Australia: Elsevier.

Kibe, L. W., & Cawley, J. F. (2018). Doctoral education for physician assistants: Demand, design, and drawbacks. In G. Kayingo & V. M. Hass (Eds.), *The health professions educator: A practical guide for new and established faculty* (pp. 397-406). New York, NY: Springer Publishing Company.

National Economic & Social Rights Initiative. (2018). *Health care in the United States*. Retrieved from https://nesri.mayfirst.org/programs/health-care-in-the-united-states

National Institute on Drug Abuse. (2019). *Opioid overdose crisis*. Retrieved from https://www.drugabuse.gov/drugs-abuse/opioids/opioid-overdose-crisis

Ornstein, C. (2010, June 15). How America's hospitals survived the first wave of the coronavirus. *ProPublica*. Retrieved from https://www.propublica.org/article/how-americas-hospitals-survived-the-first-wave-of-the-coronavirus

Palmer, K., Doig, C., & Konkin, J. (2017, July 6). Does more education for health professionals equal better patient care? Healthy Debate. Retrieved from https://healthydebate.ca/2017/07/topic/medical-education-patient-care

Rao, T. S. R., & Andrade, C. (2011). The MMR vaccine and autism: Sensation, refutation, retraction, and fraud. *Indian Journal of Psychiatry, 53*(2), 95-96. doi:10.4103/0019-5545.82529.

University of California. (2013). *A new era of growth: A closer look at recent trends in health professions education*. Retrieved from https://www.ucop.edu/uc-health/_files/a-new-era-of-growth_may2013.pdf

U.S. Department of Health and Human Services Office of Disease Prevention and Health Promotion. (n.d.). *Quick guide to health literacy*. Retrieved from https://health.gov/communication/literacy/quickguide/Quickguide.pdf

U.S. Department of Health and Human Services Office of Disease Prevention and Health Promotion. (2019a). *About healthy people*. Retrieved https://www.healthypeople.gov/2020/Abou-Healthy-People

U.S. Department of Health and Human Services Office of Disease Prevention and Health Promotion. (2019b). *Access to health services.* Retrieved from https://www.healthypeople.gov/2020/topics -objectives/topic/Access-to-Health-Services

U.S. Department of Health and Human Services Office of Disease Prevention and Health Promotion. (2019c). *Global health.* Retrieved from https://www.healthypeople.gov/2020/topics-objectives /topic/global-health

U.S. Department of Health and Human Services Office of Disease Prevention and Health Promotion. (2019d). *Health communication and health information technology.* Retrieved from https://www .healthypeople.gov/2020/topics-objectives

U.S. Department of Health and Human Services Office of Disease Prevention and Health Promotion. (2019e). *Injury and violence prevention.* Retrieved from https://www.healthypeople.gov/2020/ topics-objectives/topic/injury-and-violence-prevention

U.S. Department of Health and Human Services Office of Disease Prevention and Health Promotion. (2019f). *Lesbian, gay, bisexual, and transgender health.* Retrieved from https://www.healthypeople .gov/2020/topics-objectives/topic/lesbian-gay-bisexual-and-transgender-health

U.S. Department of Health and Human Services Office of Disease Prevention and Health Promotion. (2019g). *Older adults.* Retrieved from https://www.healthypeople.gov/2020/topics-objectives/ topic/older-adults

U.S. Department of Health and Human Services Office of Disease Prevention and Health Promotion. (2019h). *Social determinants of health.* Retrieved from https://www.healthypeople.gov/2020/topics -objectives/topic/social-determinants-of-health

U.S. Department of Labor's Bureau of Labor Statistics. (2019). *Occupational outlook handbook.* Retrieved from https://www.bls.gov/ooh/

3

Contemporary Issues in Higher Education

Much like Chapter 2, there are countless topics I could have included in this chapter, but I had to focus on a handful of issues that I felt would be most helpful for new and aspiring faculty in understanding the complex landscape of higher education. Although not every topic in this chapter will be directly relevant to you, each topic is likely important to some of your colleagues, your profession, and your institution. My goal with this chapter is to help you understand how your faculty role relates to the larger contexts of your institution and the higher education system. The sections in this chapter provide only a brief overview of some very important topics. You will learn more through experience, and you will begin to figure out which issues deserve more exploration on your part.

FUNDING IN HIGHER EDUCATION

In Chapter 4, you will learn more about the difference between public institutions, which receive state appropriations, and private institutions, which are funded by nonprofit or for-profit organizations outside of state government. Regardless of institutional type, money is always an important issue. However, this section focuses on funding issues specific to public institutions. Brown, Fuller, and Smith (2017) identified several pressures facing American higher education, including "diminished public support, declining federal and state revenue, increasing expenditures, dropping enrollments, growing competition, and new instructional delivery methods. At many institutions, these pressures necessitate limited or stagnant salary increases, hiring freezes, and reductions in resources" (p. 9).

Gateley, C. A. *Clinical Practice to Academia:*
A Guide for New and Aspiring Health Professions Faculty
(pp. 23-43). © 2021 Taylor & Francis Group.

During and after the Great Recession of 2007 to 2009, state legislatures made significant cuts to higher education funding. Although on the rebound, in 2017 overall state funding for public institutions was nearly $9 billion below 2008 funding levels after adjusting for inflation (Mitchell, Leachman, & Masterson, 2017).

> The funding decline has contributed to higher tuition and reduced quality on campuses as colleges have had to balance budgets by reducing faculty, limiting course offerings, and in some cases closing campuses. At a time when the benefit of a college education has never been greater, state policymakers have made going to college less affordable and less accessible to the students most in need. (Mitchell et al., 2017, p. 1)

Reduced state funding for higher education has resulted in a number of consequences for institutions and the people who work at and attend, or wish to attend, those institutions. These consequences include the following:

- Higher tuition for students and families
- Reduced faculty, programs, and student services
- Fewer institutional scholarships
- Concern for lack of campus diversity because students of color are less likely to enroll in college as tuition rises
- A push of lower-income students toward less selective institutions, which in turn is related to lower future earning potential

You might think that decreased funding has resulted in decreased enrollment. On the contrary, college enrollment actually rose rapidly during the recession, "particularly at community colleges, as many high school graduates chose college over dim employment prospects and older workers returned to retool and gain new skills" (Mitchell et al., 2017, p. 10).

Since the recession, federal financial aid has increased, although federal grants and loans are often not enough for students to cover the cost of tuition and other educational expenses (Mitchell et al., 2017). Additionally, state-based financial aid has steadily shifted from need-based to merit-based aid. Need-based aid is based on a student's demonstrated financial need. Merit-based aid is based on academic achievement, including high school grades and college entrance exam scores. "The growth of merit-based grants as a share of state-funded aid has created concern that they disproportionately go to students who would likely attend college anyway and, on average, shift limited state resources away from lower-income students" (Mitchell et al., 2017, p. 20).

As you explore faculty positions or begin employment at an institution, you should learn more about changes in funding over the past several years and how your institution has handled those challenges. Has tuition risen? Have there been cuts to programs, faculty, or staff? How were those decisions made? How have these changes impacted enrollment at the institution? Have there been any significant changes to the diversity of the student population that can be traced back to changes in funding and financial aid?

GLOBALIZATION OF HIGHER EDUCATION

"Higher education is increasingly a global enterprise, in just about every facet of what colleges and universities do" (Inside Higher Ed, 2014). Institutions want to recruit international students, not only to increase the diversity of their student populations but also to benefit from the tuition dollars that international students bring with them. Students and their families want more opportunities for international study abroad and internship opportunities to help prepare students to work with diverse populations in their future careers.

What does all this mean for health professions programs? Faculty and administrators must consider if and how to recruit international students to their programs. What requirements will they establish for language competency, previous degrees, or prerequisite coursework for international students applying to their programs? How will they establish opportunities for international student experiences? How do accreditation standards affect those decisions? These are just a few of the issues that health professions faculty and administrators are facing with the globalization of higher education.

TECHNOLOGY IN HIGHER EDUCATION

Over the past few decades, the changes in technology as they relate to higher education are simply remarkable. My own students look dumbfounded as I explain to them that I began college in the early 1990s with a Brother electronic typewriter (the fancy one with four different colored pens) and eventually transitioned to a word processor. I did not own a computer in college, and on the rare occasions when I had to use one, there were a few available in the library for student use. A few computer labs were just beginning to emerge across campus. My instructors used overhead projectors and transparencies, and students were required to write notes by hand. We even had to go to the library to locate books and articles for research projects. Today's college students do not remember a time without laptops, cell phones, and countless technological gadgets and programs for quickly locating and sharing information.

Technology in higher education today includes presentation software, learning management systems, student response systems, virtual reality and other simulation programs, curriculum mapping, lecture capture, online discussion boards, videoconferencing, file sharing, and countless other innovations. Multak (2018) identified the following benefits of educational technology:

- Students remain focused for longer periods of time as they use technology for exploration.
- Technology promotes active learning and stimulates excitement about learning.
- Technology allows students to engage with material at their own pace.
- The integration of technology with learning helps students develop critical thinking and work skills they will need for future success.

Unless you very recently have been a student yourself, you may be unfamiliar with the latest technology used in higher education. You need to determine if there is an instructional technology or educational technology division on your campus. Explore the resources offered. Which learning management system does the campus use? Are there trainings for new faculty? Talk to your department chair and colleagues to find out which resources you should learn more about. However, do not rely solely on the advice of established colleagues. Faculty who have been around the longest may be least open to technological changes or perhaps the least likely to have time to learn about new educational technology. As a new faculty member eager to learn as much as I could about anything that would help me be a better instructor, I was often the one willing to attend trainings and workshops and bring back new ideas to the department. Now, more than 10 years into my faculty role with more responsibilities and less free time, I occasionally find myself thinking that the resources I use are sufficient or that I do not have time to learn or incorporate something new into my courses. Luckily, I am surrounded by newer colleagues who are eager to attend those trainings and share ideas with the rest of us. Even as you advance in your faculty career, you should continually learn about and incorporate new technology into your teaching.

DISTANCE EDUCATION

Closely related to the advancements in educational technology is the proliferation of distance education. "The teaching-learning process is no longer bound by geography or conventional time constraints" (Multak, 2018, p. 87). Distance education dates back to the 1800s when higher education institutions in Europe and the United States allowed students to take courses via mail correspondence (White, 2018). Today, students can take courses and sometimes complete entire degree programs online without ever setting foot on a college campus. If you are responsible for teaching an online course, there are numerous considerations. Is the course entirely online, or is it presented in a blended format with part of the content online and part of the content in a traditional classroom setting? Is the course provided synchronously, where students receive content together in real time, or asynchronously, where they can access course material at any time that works for their schedules? An advantage to synchronous learning is that students can interact with one another and ask the instructor questions as material is presented. Many health professions programs have satellite campuses where students at multiple locations can see the instructor via video and audio link. Of course, any time technology is involved, there is the potential for technology to fail. In addition to unexpected technological glitches, if you are recording lectures or demonstrations, you need to consider the physical design of the classroom, the placement of cameras and microphones, ambient noise, and whether you can move around the classroom or need to stay in one location to remain on camera (White, 2018).

HIGHER EDUCATION IN A PANDEMIC

As mentioned briefly in Chapter 2, I originally finished this manuscript several months before the onset of the COVID-19 pandemic. Now as I write these words in mid-June 2020, higher education as we knew it has been changed in unimaginable ways, and issues like technology and distance education are at the forefront of every higher education discussion. In March, over the course of a few days, we went from tentative suggestions from administrators via email to begin considering how to transition some coursework to an online format to emergency faculty meetings, campus closures, and a full transition to online learning. On a Wednesday morning in early March, I stood in front of my class of occupational therapy students and told them that I anticipated that the remainder of the semester would look much different than originally anticipated and that we still had more questions than answers. At that point my students, mostly in their early to mid-20s, had been paying little attention to the news and were shocked at what I was telling them. "When do you think it might happen?" they asked incredulously. I told them that I thought our institution hoped to make it through the following week, which would have been right before the scheduled Spring Break. The announcement for cancellation of all in-person classes came 6 hours later, and I never saw my students in person again.

Faculty across the United States were suddenly faced with the challenge of trying to figure out how to teach their students from a distance in the middle of a pandemic that turned life as we knew it upside down. There are countless issues related to this, far too many to address adequately in a few brief paragraphs, but I would like to share some of my own challenges, responses, and observations from the past few months. First, I very quickly had to learn how to use Zoom, the chosen video conferencing platform at my university. I previously had been an occasional participant in Zoom meetings set up by others, perhaps for an out-of-state interview during our application process, but I had never scheduled or hosted a Zoom meeting. I participated in several trainings offered through my campus and found additional online trainings to learn all the features that would increase student interaction. I also sought out trainings and self-tutorials on VoiceThread, Panopto, Flipgrid, and several other ways to share information with students and increase student engagement and interaction. Faculty within my department and across our school and institution shared ideas with each other. I joined a few social media groups whose focus is higher education distance learning, and while scrolling through the many stories of frustration, I still occasionally find a useful strategy that I can incorporate in my own courses.

Now early into the Summer 2020 semester, I am becoming much more adept with the various online teaching and learning tools and strategies, and the students are slowly adapting to the changes. However, the consistent message I am hearing from them is that online learning is hard! They have a mix of synchronous and asynchronous content across their courses, and many of them are struggling with the lack of daily structure of going to class and interacting with their faculty and peers. Particularly in most health professions programs, the students did not sign up to be online learners, and we faculty did not sign up to be online instructors. Yet, here we are, making the best of the situation we find ourselves in. Sometimes I make mistakes and forget to "publish" a document in the learning management system or to "share" my screen in Zoom so students can view what I am talking about. Sometimes they make mistakes and forget to hit "submit" on a timed online quiz. Without lowering my expectations of what they need to learn and the competencies they need to demonstrate, I have certainly become much more understanding of student issues like inconsistently reliable technology and challenges with assignment submission.

As we prepare for the 2020–2021 academic year, none of us really knows what to expect. Like many institutions across the country, mine currently plans to resume in-person classes, although the degree to which that can occur remains to be seen (Burke, 2020). We have been asked to decide what percentage of each course absolutely needs to be taught in person and what can be transitioned to online or blended learning. We have to consider bringing students in for several small lab groups throughout the day to maintain social distancing rather than having nearly 50 people packed into a crowded classroom at once, which subsequently creates staffing, space, and scheduling issues. We have to plan for the personal protective equipment and screening strategies that will be needed for students, faculty, and other classroom and lab participants, such as clients and guest presenters, to safely be in each other's presence. We have to figure out creative ways to schedule students for the mandatory fieldwork experiences to meet our profession's accreditation guidelines at a time when no facility wants extra germ-carriers entering their buildings. Meanwhile, our campus is facing a budget crisis related to massive cuts in state funding and projected shortfalls in student enrollment. Faculty and staff across our academic health system are facing layoffs, furloughs, salary cuts, and job or program elimination.

My institution's situation is not unique. Every higher education institution is facing some kind of unprecedented challenge. Yuen (2020) claimed "the coronavirus pandemic has led to the most difficult semester in generations on college campuses across the United States" (para. 1). I agree that this pandemic and its aftermath is the most significant threat to higher education any of us have ever seen. I hope that by the time many of you read these words, the pandemic will be old news and higher education will be back on the upswing! Whether or not that occurs, there are many lessons to be learned from this situation regarding adaptability and the obligation of faculty to do their best for students no matter the situation.

INTERPROFESSIONAL EDUCATION

In 2010, the World Health Organization published the *Framework for Action on Interprofessional Education and Collaborative Practice.* The World Health Organization explained that interprofessional education "occurs when two or more professions learn about, from and with each other to enable effective collaboration and improve health outcomes" (2010, p. 13). Interprofessional education has gained considerable attention and buy-in from health professions educational programs over the past decade. The Interprofessional Education Collaborative (IPEC) was established in 2009 to promote interprofessional learning experiences with initial efforts focused on medicine, nursing, pharmacy, dentistry, and public health. By 2017, numerous health and other professions had become members of the IPEC, including nutrition and dietetics, physical therapy, occupational therapy, psychology, speech-language and hearing, social work, and physician assistants (IPEC, 2018). If you are a new or aspiring health professions faculty member, explore the initiatives currently underway by your institution and profession.

DIVERSITY AND INCLUSION OF STUDENTS

We often hear the terms *diversity* and *inclusion* lumped together in a single phrase, but they hold separate meanings. The Ferris State University Diversity Office (n.d.) explains this as follows:

> Diversity is the range of human differences, including but not limited to race, ethnicity, gender, gender identity, sexual orientation, age, social class, physical ability or attributes, religious or ethical values system, national origin, and political beliefs. Inclusion is involvement and empowerment, where the inherent worth and dignity of all people are recognized. An inclusive university promotes and sustains a sense of belonging; it values and practices respect for the talents, beliefs, backgrounds, and ways of living of its members. (para. 1)

The U.S. population is more diverse than ever before and so are the students entering higher education institutions. However, there continue to be racial and ethnic disparities in higher education application, admission, enrollment, persistence, and degree completion (U.S. Department of Education, Office of Planning, Evaluation and Policy Development and Office of the Under Secretary, 2016). Health professions programs are not immune to this. In my own program, despite recruitment efforts and recent implementation of a more holistic admissions process, approximately 90% of students accepted into our highly competitive program over the past decade were White. Students of color who do gain entrance into health professions programs face additional challenges. "Because of education inequities [at the K–12 level], when students from underrepresented backgrounds and underserved communities seek health professions education, they often have a variety of learning needs that, thus far, health professions educators have been underprepared to meet" (Ackerman-Barger, Acosta, Bakerjian, Murray-Garcia, & Ton, 2018, p. 224).

If you are seeking a faculty position or have recently accepted one, you should explore how these issues affect your institution and your specific program. What are the demographic trends for application, admission, enrollment, persistence, and degree completion? Does your program or institution have any strategic priorities related to diversity, inclusion, and equity in student outcomes? How are administrators addressing those issues? What will be your role as a faculty member in addressing those issues?

MINORITY FACULTY

Just as there are inequities in the number of students who enter and graduate from health professions programs, so, too, are there disparities in the number of minority faculty entering and remaining in health professions programs. Reasons for attrition include racism, sexism, experiences of marginalization, and a phenomenon known as the *diversity tax* or *diversity burden* in which "minority faculty are often expected to go above and beyond other faculty by mentoring and advising minority students, teaching topics related to diversity (whether related to their area of expertise or not), and representing diversity on initiatives and in committees" (Mulitalo, Ackerman-Barger, Ryujin, & Lund, 2018, p. 238). Furthermore, faculty of color who work at institutions that are predominantly White may encounter overt hostility; subtle expressions of prejudice or bias; and "unconscious racism, classism, and elitism toward minority group faculty colleagues or minority studies or students by otherwise well-intentioned mainstream faculty" (McKay, 2007, p. 67).

If you are an individual from a minority background who is seeking an academic position, look for institutions and programs that have a stated commitment to inclusion in their mission statements, strategic plans, and other documents. Are there entities in place at the school or campus level that specifically address these issues, such as an office of diversity and inclusion or office of equity and inclusion? How many other minority faculty exist in the program, school, or across campus? Are there programs in place to connect you with other minority faculty for support and mentorship? If you are not from a minority background, you should still be concerned with these issues. What value does your institution and program place on diversity and inclusion? What practices are in place to improve the campus experience for your colleagues of color? How can you contribute to those efforts?

WOMEN IN ACADEMIA

Scholars have been researching and writing about women in academia for decades. A cursory review of that literature brings up several important issues. "Women continue to be underrepresented in academe, particularly at the highest ranks, and those who do enter the professional academic world may be subjected to a host of sexist attitudes and practices" (Moe & Murphy, 2011, p. 60). Although illegal, inquiries about personal lives often come up in conversations during the interview process, perhaps suggesting concern that women will put personal issues ahead of professional endeavors.

Another concern is the persistent pay gap between men and women in faculty and administrative positions in higher education. Data from the 2017 to 2018 annual Faculty Compensation Survey published by the American Association of University Professors (AAUP) indicate that "93 percent of all participating institutions pay men more than women at the same rank" (Flaherty, 2018). However, this statistic is based on aggregate data that do not discern factors such as discipline or length of service at a particular rank. Toth (2007) noted the following: "Although the pay gap in academia persists, it is smaller than the gap in other professions" (p. 61).

Beyond inequities in employment and compensation, women in higher education "may be subjected to gendered expectations with regard to particular types of service" such as organizing events and advising students (Moe & Murphy, 2011, p. 63). These expectations may come from both colleagues and students, "with students feeling more comfortable coming to female faculty about their concerns, and exhibiting greater informality in doing so" (Moe & Murphy, 2011, p. 63).

Although these issues are certainly relevant for many women in higher education, they are not a significant part of my own experience as a faculty member. Perhaps I have a skewed perception because my profession, like many health professions, is female-dominated, or maybe it is because I have a department chair who consistently makes sure faculty in our department know that his expectation is always "family first, work second." Across my department and my school of health professions, the majority of faculty are women, and I believe my salary is on par with my male colleagues. Do students come to me and my female colleagues with academic and personal concerns more frequently than my male colleagues? Probably so, but I have never felt like this expectation was forced on me by male colleagues and administrators. Are males disproportionately represented in administrative positions across my school such as program director, department chair, or dean? I honestly do not know. I also do not know if any women applied for those positions when they were open or what their qualifications may have been in relation to the men who ended up in those administrative positions.

These are all tough but important issues to think about as you consider a career as a health professions faculty member. Toth (2007) suggested that new female faculty members should find themselves female mentors. Additionally, Toth recommended "a new woman faculty member should join whatever women's faculty groups exist: whatever her field, she'll almost certainly need them. She needs a support system: women who'll tell her honestly what goes on at a university, for women" (p. 51).

LEGAL ISSUES IN HIGHER EDUCATION

The Family Educational Rights and Privacy Act

Coming from a health professions background, you undoubtedly have heard of the Health Insurance Portability and Accountability Act of 1996 and subsequent legislation, which mandate the privacy and protection of personal health information (U.S. Department of Health & Human Services, 2013). Unless you previously worked in an educational setting, you may be less familiar with the Family Educational Rights and Privacy Act (FERPA), which protects the rights of student education records (U.S. Department of Education, n.d.). The rights to educational records transfer to students when they turn 18 or enroll in education beyond the high school level. This means that, unless the student provides written or electronic consent, parents of college students do not have access to their students' academic records or the bills associated with their enrollment. As I will discuss more in Chapter 9, many parents of today's college students are used to managing every aspect of their children's lives, so the sudden lack of access and control once their students reach college does not always go over well. Having experienced two different college orientation sessions with my own daughters over the past few years, I have witnessed my fair share of angry and incredulous parents, all with the same message—"I'm paying the bill. What do you mean I can't look at the grades?!" Many institutions have made efforts to educate parents about FERPA and include them more in the orientation and transition process to help reduce such frustrations and encourage partnerships between institutions and parents (Cutright, 2008).

So, what does FERPA mean for you? Most campuses will have a required annual training for faculty and staff clearly outlining what your responsibilities and restrictions are in terms of sharing information about your students. I personally have had very few instances of parents seeking information about their students, but my experience is primarily in graduate- and professional-level programs at a large research institution. I know colleagues who teach at the undergraduate level and in other institutional types who have story after story about parents getting involved in their college students' academic issues. If you encounter any requests for information regarding a student's academic performance, refer to your institution's FERPA training materials or ask an administrator for guidance.

Title IX

In addition to FERPA, if you are seeking a faculty position, you need to understand Title IX of the Education Amendments of 1972, typically referred to as Title IX, which states the following: "No person in the United States shall, on the basis of sex, be excluded from participation in, be denied the benefits of, or be subjected to discrimination under any education program or activity receiving Federal financial assistance" (U.S. Department of Education, Office for Civil Rights, 2015, para. 2).

I had heard of Title IX before I began in my faculty role, but I thought it had only to do with institutions having an equal number of athletic opportunities for men and women. I know now that Title IX includes not just athletics but also academics, extracurricular activities, and employment (Weniger & Knight, 2018). Title IX protects students, employees, and applicants for admission or employment from all forms of sex discrimination. This means your academic program cannot treat students or applicants differently based on their gender or gender identity when making admissions decisions or determining clinical assignments.

The part that surprised me most when I learned more about Title IX is that I am a mandated reporter if I have reason to believe that any student at my institution has experienced student-on-student sexual violence. If a student discloses to me that he or she was raped at a party, I am required by law to report it to the Title IX coordinator on campus, even if the student begs for confidentiality. If I inadvertently overhear students talking about an incident of sexual violence before or after class, I am required to report it to the Title IX coordinator. The only exceptions to this mandatory responsibility are "mental-health counselors, pastoral counselors, social workers, psychologists, health center employees, or any other person with a professional license requiring confidentiality, or who is supervised by such a person" (U.S. Department of Education, Office for

Civil Rights, n.d., p. 22). Your campus should have an office that investigates reports of Title IX violations, and you may be required to complete periodic training regarding your responsibilities as a campus employee.

UNDERSTANDING VARIOUS FACULTY TYPES

When I began my college teaching career, I had very little understanding of the different types of faculty positions in higher education. I know now that there are various academic titles across my institution, each with different responsibilities and expectations. I also know that faculty titles and expectations vary greatly across institutional types. This section provides a brief overview of some of the most common faculty classifications.

Tenured and Tenure-Track Faculty

Tenure refers to an indefinite appointment granted to a faculty member after a long probationary status (Finkin, 2007). Aspects of the tenure system can be traced back centuries through world history. In the United States, tenure arose in the decades after the Civil War when the following occurred:

> Colleges and universities began adopting the German higher education model, which emphasized science and research.... With the growth of this research university model, American professors began to expect the same perks that their German colleagues enjoyed, including indefinite appointments except in cases of gross dereliction of duty. (Harris, 2018, para. 1)

In 1915, the AAUP was founded, and members sought protections for faculty members after several instances of faculty being fired for presenting views that were not consistent with popular opinion. In 1940, the AAUP and the Association of American Colleges and Universities jointly published the *Statement of Principles on Academic Freedom and Tenure,* which remains a guiding document across higher education (Harris, 2018). Once a faculty member achieves tenure, he or she can only be terminated under extraordinary circumstances. "The principal purpose of tenure is to safeguard academic freedom, which is necessary for all who teach and conduct research in higher education" (AAUP, n.d., para. 3). In other words, tenure protects a faculty member from being fired for something he or she says, researches, or publishes. The AAUP asserts that tenure also serves the public interest.

> Education and research benefit society, but society does not benefit when teachers and researchers are controlled by corporations, religious groups, special interest groups, or the government. Free inquiry, free expression, and open dissent are critical for student learning and the advancement of knowledge. Therefore, it is important to have systems in place to protect academic freedom. Tenure serves that purpose. (AAUP, n.d., para. 4)

The tenure process varies by institutional type. I teach at a large, public, research institution where new tenure-track faculty typically are hired at the assistant professor level, and they are expected to be productive in scholarly endeavors, such as grant-funded research and publications. Teaching and service are also part of their expectations, but scholarly productivity often is most heavily valued in the tenure process at research institutions. Krieger (2013) explained that other institutional types may have different expectations for tenure-track faculty that place more emphasis on the faculty member's teaching and service contributions. At the end of 5 years, tenure-track faculty submit a dossier detailing their various academic accomplishments.

The dossier undergoes review by faculty peers and administrators at various levels (i.e., department, school, and campus) who determine whether the individual will be granted tenure and promoted to the rank of associate professor. If the quantity and quality of work are not deemed worthy of tenure, the individual instead is given a 1-year terminal appointment and must seek employment elsewhere. Many institutions also have a third-year review process for tenure-track faculty. Peers and administrators review the faculty member's dossier at the end of the third year of employment to determine if the individual is on track to achieve tenure. If there is concern for poor scholarly performance and productivity, the individual may be granted a 1-year terminal contract at that time.

Faculty who previously were granted tenure and the rank of associate professor may submit a dossier for consideration of promotion to the rank of full professor after at least another 5 years. Some institutions do not award tenure until a faculty member has achieved the rank of professor (Krieger, 2013). Depending on prior experience and accomplishments, some faculty initially are hired with tenure at the rank of associate professor or professor.

As you can imagine, *going up for tenure*, as the process is often called, is a long and often anxiety-ridden process for faculty. The prospect of being denied tenure and needing to secure a faculty position at another institution or consider other career paths is not pleasant. The reality is that some faculty achieve tenure, whereas others do not. Simply putting in 5 years of work and submitting a dossier will not earn you tenure and promotion. Your work has to be at the level expected for your institution, as viewed through the eyes of the specific individuals involved in the review of your dossier. The standards for promotion and tenure may change over time, and those changes may be either explicit or implicit (Krieger, 2013). Again, every institution has its own hiring, tenure, and promotion policies, and you should become familiar with the policies and processes at your institution. "Keep in mind that the university tenure and promotion guidelines are meant to help the university make its faculty stronger, and make the process fair and more transparent" (Krieger, 2013, p. 227).

Non–Tenure-Track Faculty

Although it was the norm at many U.S. institutions for decades, the tenure system has shrunk considerably in recent years. By 2016, the percentage of instructional positions not on the tenure track was 73% across all institutional types combined (AAUP, 2018). "The increase in contingent faculty happened due to the combination of unprecedented growth in student enrollment, administrative misjudgments of that growth, and decline in government funding and public support of higher education." (Kezar, 2012b, p. xi). The AAUP, an organization whose mission in part is to maintain quality higher education and preserve academic freedom, views the shift away from the tenure system as a negative trend.

> For the most part, these are insecure, unsupported positions with little job security and few protections of academic freedom. Depending on the institution, contingent faculty can be known as adjuncts, postdocs, TAs, non-tenure-track faculty, clinical faculty, part-timers, lecturers, instructors, or non-senate faculty. (AAUP, 2018, p. 1)

I should make clear here that this description has, for the most part, not been my experience as a full-time, non–tenure-track (NTT) faculty member. I teach in a health profession that has high market demand and, therefore, high demand for educational programs and qualified faculty and administrators to lead those programs. I have never felt significant concern about job security. However, I have witnessed the elimination of NTT faculty positions across my school and campus during periods of economic downturn and decreased state funding. I have also heard stories from NTT faculty in my profession who teach at other institutions where they experience these concerns to a much higher degree. In the following subsections, I discuss some of the concerns for two distinct groups of NTT faculty, those who are employed on a full-time basis and those who are employed on a part-time or adjunct basis.

Full-Time Non–Tenure-Track Faculty

Full-time NTT faculty typically have salaried positions with short-term contracts that may be semester to semester or year to year (Kezar, 2012b). "The status of pedagogically oriented faculty is gradually increasing at research-intensive universities, as administrators are coming to appreciate their educational contributions and are responding with improved status, greater job security, and higher salaries" (Gross & Goldenberg, 2007, p. 146). At my institution, NTT faculty who have achieved the rank of associate NTT professor or NTT professor have the potential to receive 3- or 5-year contracts, respectively.

If you are seeking a full-time NTT position, you should explore the following issues before applying and throughout the interview and orientation process (Kezar, 2012a):

- How does the institution define academic roles? Is there "a system of sequential ranks and opportunities for salary increases?" (Kezar, 2012a, p. 7)
- How are NTT faculty evaluated for reappointment?
- What opportunities exist for professional development? Is there funding to attend professional development opportunities on or off campus?
- Are there opportunities for recognition or awards for excellence in teaching and service, two primary responsibilities of NTT faculty?
- Are NTT faculty involved in faculty governance? According to Kezar (2012a, p. 8), "A long-held characteristic of professionals is their involvement in creating their conditions of work and impacting the larger work environment."
- Are there any campus committees specifically for NTT faculty?
- Is there adequate office space, clerical support, and equipment for NTT faculty to perform their work, meet with students, and prepare for teaching?

An issue that came up when I recently served on a campus-level NTT task force was how NTT faculty are labeled. One committee member did not like the term *non–tenure-track faculty*. He argued that "We should be defined by who we are, not by who we are not." Institutions may also use terms such as *fixed term, limited term, lecturer, instructor*, or *contingent faculty*. Hoikkala (2012) stated that "contingency often implies an internalized sense of inferiority" among NTT faculty (p. 130). Hoikkala further explained that NTT faculty are sometimes described as apathetic. "What is often labeled apathy is really just a deep sense of powerlessness, an internalized feeling of inability to change what is" (Hoikkala, 2012, p. 131). Whalen (2012) explained that when NTT faculty are appropriately valued by their tenured and tenure-track colleagues, they have the opportunity "to become truly integrated members of the faculty" (p. 151).

I have been a full-time NTT faculty member for over 10 years. I have always felt valued by colleagues and administrators within my own department and school of health professions. I have had the opportunity for promotion and recognition for teaching excellence. However, I have been frustrated at times by campus policies and procedures that obviously place higher emphasis on research than teaching. I teach at a research-intensive institution, so I certainly understand the emphasis on research. My institution is also a member of the American Association of Universities (AAU), an elite group of 62 research universities that "earn the majority of competitively awarded federal funding for research that improves public health, seeks to address national challenges, and contributes significantly to our economic strength, while educating and training tomorrow's visionary leaders and innovators" (AAU, n.d., para. 1). This prestigious distinction is part of my institution's identity, but at times the emphasis on maintaining AAU membership leaves some NTT faculty feeling less valued. For example, certain aspects of annual performance reviews are designed to capture the scholarly productivity of faculty in terms of the number and monetary value of external grants, research publications, the prestige of journals in which research was published, and several other factors that may be completely irrelevant for an NTT faculty member who has little or no expectation of scholarly productivity. I have been disheartened to complete these mandatory annual forms, which ultimately make it look as though I accomplished nothing in comparison to my tenured and tenure-track colleagues.

In summary, if you are seeking a full-time NTT faculty position, ask about the issues discussed earlier. More specifically, ask other NTT faculty about these issues because they may have very different perceptions than tenured and tenure-track faculty. It is important to understand the culture of the institution and understand how NTT faculty are valued as part of the overall academic community.

Part-Time and Adjunct Non–Tenure-Track Faculty

Many NTT faculty are hired on a part-time or adjunct basis to teach one or two courses. This is how I began my transition into academia. In 2007, a faculty member from my alma mater contacted me to see if I would be interested in teaching a course in pediatric occupational therapy because the department was in a period of transition and had not yet hired a full-time faculty member to take over teaching the course. Having recently considered a transition to college teaching, I jumped at the opportunity, with absolutely no idea what I was doing. I was given the previous syllabus and textbook and a small amount of guidance and then was set free to plan a course that would begin less than 3 weeks later. I was not given any training in the learning management system. In fact, I had no idea one even existed until midway through the semester when a student asked, "Why don't you just put everything on Blackboard for us?" To accommodate the schedule of my full-time clinical job, I taught the course in the evenings, so I rarely saw any of the other faculty or support staff. If I wanted any handouts copied for class, I had to make arrangements to drop the originals with the administrative assistant the week before and hope that they got left in a location I could access the following week. If I needed Internet access, I had to ask another faculty member or a student to log in to the classroom computer for me. I did not have office space to do work preparation or meet with students. I was unaware of campus supports that may have been useful to an adjunct faculty member. Did I impart some knowledge and skills to that first cohort of students I taught? I would like to think so. Would I do a much better job if I had the opportunity to redo that semester? Absolutely.

Although support for adjunct faculty has improved considerably within my own department over the past decade, my experience as an adjunct faculty member for one semester is not unusual. "Upon hire, adjuncts frequently find themselves without access to some of the basic resources they need to adequately perform their job," such as office space, library privileges, sample syllabi, and curriculum guidelines (Brown et al., 2017, p. 22). In a recent survey of adjunct faculty developers, Smith and Fuller (2017) reported that some individuals "described institutions that treated adjunct faculty as second-class members of the college or university" (p. 77). "For many adjuncts, the working conditions are brutal and position them in a lower tier than full-time [NTT faculty] and tenured and tenure-track faculty" (Hensley, 2017, p. 44).

Adjunct faculty are often hired to teach courses when enrollment exceeds the capacity of full-time faculty to teach courses. The use of adjunct faculty is rapidly increasing across higher education. "Adjunct faculty now compose the largest single category of educators in the higher education workforce, constituting approximately 50% of all college faculty" (Brown et al., 2017, p. 11). Building on the work of previous scholars, Brown et al. (2017) proposed the following typology of adjunct or part-time faculty:

- Voluntary part-time faculty:
  - Graduate students: For some graduate students, serving as a teaching assistant may be required as part of their financial aid package, stipend, or tuition waiver. Others may want to gain experience because they hope to obtain full-time faculty roles in the future.
  - Outside specialists: These are experts within a particular field who are recruited or seek out teaching opportunities in their discipline. I imagine this category is the one in which many of the readers of this book fall.
  - Voluntary freelancers: These individuals combine part-time teaching with other part-time employment. Health care professionals who either cannot find or do not want a full-time faculty position may fall into this category. Perhaps they teach a few courses and maintain part-time clinical employment as well.
  - Career enders: These individuals have retired from full-time careers, possibly even full-time academic careers, but they desire to keep current with their profession and to teach the next generation of practitioners for their profession.
- Involuntary part-time faculty:
  - Aspiring hopefuls: These individuals recently completed a degree, and part-time teaching was the best opportunity available. I would argue that many health professions faculty may be included here as well. They have decided to make the transition to full-time teaching, but they have not yet obtained a full-time position.
  - Involuntary freelancers: These individuals combine multiple part-time teaching positions at multiple institutions because full-time positions are not available. I know a few colleagues in my own profession who live in urban areas and work at two or three different institutions to piece together the equivalent of full-time work without the benefits associated with a full-time salaried position, such as health care and retirement plans.

Kezar (2017) expressed concern that "the isolation of adjunct faculty contributes not only to their job satisfaction but also to their ability to advance as professionals and to partake in a professional community" (p. xi). Many institutions are beginning to recognize the importance of doing a better job of training and supporting the adjunct faculty who are teaching so many of their students. "If institutions are going to employ adjunct faculty, they need to have structures in place to ensure that adjunct faculty are able to demonstrate excellence in their service to students and the rest of the institution" (Smith & Fuller, 2017, p. 80). The following are examples of initiatives by various institutions to provide professional development opportunities for adjunct faculty:

- Kirkwood Community College in Iowa has an Adjunct Faculty Advisory Committee. The institution also provides an orientation program, ongoing support, and inclusion in campus communications, and conducts an annual survey of adjunct faculty (Bonde, 2017).

- Saginaw Valley State University in Michigan has an Office of Adjunct Faculty Support Programs, an adjunct faculty handbook, training in the campus learning management system, training regarding teaching fundamentals and classroom management skills, and ongoing professional development opportunities for adjunct faculty (Coburn-Collins, Acker, Altevogt, & Tsay, 2017).
- GateWay Community College in Arizona established an Adjunct Faculty Academy, which provides an overview of pedagogy and curriculum design, connects adjunct faculty with campus resources and other adjuncts, and provides networking opportunities for adjuncts who are seeking full-time employment on the campus (Cherland, Crook, Dippold, Gabardiel, & Remy, 2017).
- A social work program at an anonymous research university developed a department-specific orientation for adjunct faculty. The program also assists them with syllabus development; connects them with other faculty; and provides part-time teaching assistant support, brown-bag lunches, evening trainings on teaching skills, and awards to recognize excellence in adjunct teaching (Fagan, 2017).

These are just a few of the examples across the country of how institutions are supporting adjunct faculty. If you are considering an adjunct faculty position, ask what type of orientation and ongoing support you will have. Find out if there is a center for teaching and learning that offers professional development opportunities. Are those opportunities available at a time that will work for your adjunct schedule? Shropshire (2017) emphasized the importance of adjunct faculty members finding a mentor on the campus that they can turn to when they have questions or need guidance. Putman and Kriner (2017) encouraged adjunct faculty to seek out communities of practice (i.e., groups of people with common goals of professional development) to help learn best teaching practices and to reduce feelings of isolation among adjunct faculty.

FACULTY SALARIES

Each year, the AAUP conducts a Faculty Compensation Survey, which is "the largest independent source of data on full-time faculty salary and benefits at two- and four-year colleges and universities in the United States" (Inside Higher Ed, 2019). Data from the survey are summarized in the "Annual Report on the Economic Status of the Profession," which is published each year in *Academe*, the AAUP's magazine. The report includes narrative summaries about issues such as gender-based disparities, salary compression, medical and retirement benefits, and economic prospects for faculty. The data are also presented in an easily searchable database at www.insidehighered.com

Beyond the national data on faculty salaries, you may be able to locate salary information for your specific institution, particularly if it is a public institution. Try an online search using the name of the institution in combination with keywords such as "faculty salaries" or "salary database." You should be able to locate a database in which you can then search by using either your profession as a keyword or by searching for specific names of individuals you know are employed there. Keep in mind as you browse the salary information that those individuals have been at the institution for varying lengths of time and may have various titles and responsibilities that affect their salaries. You cannot expect to start out making the same salary as someone who has been at the institution for 12 years and has been promoted multiple times.

LEARNING ACTIVITIES

1. Which topics in this chapter are most relevant to you at this point in your career? Why? What other resources can you locate to learn more about these issues?

2. Explore the funding sources for an institution of interest to you. Is it publicly or privately funded? Are there any recent news stories about funding or budget issues for the institution?

3. Look for information about how globalization affects your profession, institution, and department. Are there study-abroad programs or international experiences for students? What involvement do faculty have in those programs?

4. Explore the educational technology available at your institution. What learning management system is used for courses? What training is available for faculty? Is there an educational technology division or center? What other trainings are offered that may be useful to a new faculty member?

5. Does your department offer any coursework online? What support can you find for faculty who teach distance education courses? Look at campus resources as well as other resources you can find online.

6. Can you locate any initiatives involving interprofessional education for your specific program? What about across your profession?

7. What evidence can you locate for your department, institution, and profession about commitment to diversity and inclusion?

8. Look for information about minority faculty in your profession and at your particular institution. Are there any groups that support and advocate for these individuals?

9. Explore the websites for your national professional association and institution. Are there any groups specific to women in academia? Are there any professional development opportunities, such as a women's leadership conference?

10. Explore the websites of one or more institutions. Look for information about FERPA and Title IX. What guidance can you locate for faculty?

11. What are the various faculty titles and ranks for your institution? You may find this type of information in the faculty handbook or a collected rules and regulations website. Each institution may have different terminology, so you may have to do some exploring to locate the relevant resources.

12. What promotion policies and procedures are in place for various faculty types? How much guidance is provided? What information should you start keeping track of for future promotion?

13. Can you locate any resources specific to NTT and adjunct faculty? Are there any professional development opportunities on your campus? If not, which other resources can you locate that would be helpful for new faculty?
14. Explore salary data for your institution. If it is a public institution, look at the salary information for faculty in your profession and other health professions. Looking at department websites, can you determine how long each person has been there and what his or her rank or position is? What trends can you identify?
15. Explore how the COVID-19 pandemic affected educational programs in your profession. How were classes and clinical experiences impacted? Talk to faculty and/or students who experienced those changes. What insights or advice do they have for you as a new or future faculty member?

REFERENCES

Ackerman-Barger, K., Acosta, D., Bakerjian, D., Murray-Garcia, J., & Ton, H. (2018). Equity pedagogy: Applying multicultural education in health professions learning environments. In G. Kayingo & V. M. Hass (Eds.), *The health professions educator: A practical guide for new and established faculty* (pp. 223-236). New York, NY: Springer Publishing Company.

American Association of Universities. (n.d.). *Who we are: About AAU*. Retrieved from https://www.aau.edu/who-we-are

American Association of University Professors. (n.d.). *Tenure*. Retrieved from https://www.aaup.org/issues/tenure

American Association of University Professors. (2018, October 11). *Data snapshot: Contingent faculty in US higher ed*. Retrieved from https://www.aaup.org/news/data-snapshot-contingent-faculty-us-higher-ed#.Xs_W_jpKhPY

Bonde, L. (2017). Creating an adjunct community and supporting its professional development: Kirkwood Community College. In R. Fuller, M. K. Brown, & K. Smith (Eds.), *Adjunct faculty voices: Cultivating professional development and community at the front lines of higher education* (pp. 98-104). Sterling, VA: Stylus.

Brown, M. K., Fuller, R., & Smith, K. (2017). A portrait of adjunct faculty. In R. Fuller, M. K. Brown, & K. Smith (Eds.), *Adjunct faculty voices: Cultivating professional development and community at the front lines of higher education* (pp. 9-36). Sterling, VA: Stylus.

Burke, L. (2020, June 9) Fall comes into view. *Inside Higher Ed.* Retrieved from https://www.insidehighered.com/news/2020/06/09/colleges-continue-announcing-plans-fall-amid-pandemic

Cherland, S., Crook, H., Dippold, L., Gabardel, J. W., & Remy, J. (2017). The transformative effects of an adjunct faculty academy: One approach to teaching adjuncts pedagogy, instructional design, and best practices. In R. Fuller, M. K. Brown, & K. Smith (Eds.), *Adjunct faculty voices: Cultivating professional development and community at the front lines of higher education* (pp. 112-118). Sterling, VA: Stylus.

Coburn-Collins, A., Acker, A. M., Altevogt, L. L., & Tsay, L. S. (2017). Cultivating scholarly teaching through professional development. In R. Fuller, M. K. Brown, & K. Smith (Eds.), *Adjunct faculty voices: Cultivating professional development and community at the front lines of higher education* (pp. 105-111). Sterling, VA: Stylus.

Cutright, M. (2008). From helicopter parent to valued partner: Shaping the parental relationship for student success. *New Directions for Higher Education, 2008*(144), 39-48.

Fagan, R. (2017). Best practices and innovative faculty development for adjunct faculty. In R. Fuller, M. K. Brown, & K. Smith (Eds.), *Adjunct faculty voices: Cultivating professional development and community at the front lines of higher education* (pp. 119-124). Sterling, VA: Stylus.

Ferris State University Diversity Office. (n.d.). *Diversity and inclusion definitions*. Retrieved from https://www.ferris.edu/HTMLS/administration/president/DiversityOffice

Finkin, M. W. (2007). The tenure system. In A. L. Deneef & C. D. Goodwin (Eds.) *The academic's handbook* (3rd ed., pp. 155-167). Durham, NC: Duke University Press.

Flaherty, C. (2018, April 11). *Faculty salaries up 3%*. Inside Higher Ed. Retrieved from https://www.insidehighered.com/news/2018/04/11/aaups-annual-report-faculty-compensation-takes-salary-compression-and-more

Gross, J. G., & Goldenberg, E. N. (2007) Off-track vetting. In A. L. Deneef & C. D. Goodwin (Eds.), *The academic's handbook* (3rd ed., pp. 144-154). Durham, NC: Duke University Press.

Harris, M. (2018, April 23). History of tenure. http://higheredprofessor.com/2018/04/23history-of-tenure

Hensley, B. (2017). Cocreating communities of adjunct faculty: Mobilizing adjunct voices through connective storytelling. In R. Fuller, M. K. Brown, & K. Smith (Eds.), *Adjunct faculty voices: Cultivating professional development and community at the front lines of higher education* (pp. 39-45). Sterling, VA: Stylus

Hoikkala, P. (2012). "Lecturers anonymous": Moving contingent faculty to visibility at a master's institution. In A. Kezar (Ed.), *Embracing non-tenure track faculty: Changing campuses for the new faculty majority* (pp. 130-145). New York, NY: Routledge.

Inside Higher Ed. (2014). *Globalization of higher education*. Retrieved from https://www.insidehighered.com/system/files/media/Globalization.pdf

Inside Higher Ed. (2019). *2017-18 AAUP Faculty Compensation Survey*. Retrieved from https://www.insidehighered.com/aaup-compensation-survey

Interprofessional Education Collaborative. (2018). *What is interprofessional education?* Retrieved from https://www.ipecollaborative.org/about-ipec.html

Kezar, A. (2012a). Needed policies, practices, and values: Creating a culture to support and professionalize non-tenure track faculty. In A. Kezar (Ed.), *Embracing non-tenure track faculty: Changing campuses for the new faculty majority* (pp. 2-27). New York, NY: Routledge.

Kezar, A. (2012b). Preface. In A. Kezar (Ed.), *Embracing non-tenure track faculty: Changing campuses for the new faculty majority* (pp. x-xxiv). New York, NY: Routledge.

Kezar, A. (2017). Foreword. In R. Fuller, M. K. Brown, & K. Smith (Eds.), *Adjunct faculty voices: Cultivating professional development and community at the front lines of higher education* (pp. xi-xiii). Sterling, VA: Stylus Publishing, LLC.

Krieger, M. H. (2013). *The scholar's survival manual*. Bloomington, IN: Indiana University Press.

McKay, N. Y. (2007). Minority faculty in [mainstream white] academia. In A. L. Deneef & C. D. Goodwin (Eds.), *The academic's handbook* (3rd ed., pp. 62-76). Durham, NC: Duke University Press.

Mitchell, M., Leachman, M., & Masterson, K. (2017, August 23). *A lost decade in higher education funding: State cuts have driven up tuition and reduced quality*. Center on Budget and Policy Priorities. Retrieved from https://www.cbpp.org/research/state-budget-and-tax/a-lost-decade-in-higher-education-funding

Moe, A. M., & Murphy, L. M. (2011). Being a new faculty. In E. Lenning, S. Brightman, & S. Caringella (Eds.), *A guide to surviving a career in academia: Navigating the rites of passage*. New York, NY: Routledge.

Mulitalo, K., Ackerman-Barger, K., Ryujin, D. T., & Lund, M. B. (2018). Minority faculty: Recruitment, retention, and advancement. In G. Kayingo & V.M. Hass (Eds.), *The health professions educator: A practical guide for new and established faculty* (pp. 237-246). New York, NY: Springer Publishing Company.

Multak, N. (2018). Technology in the classroom. In G. Kayingo & V. M. Hass (Eds.), *The health professions educator: A practical guide for new and established faculty* (pp. 87-94). New York, NY: Springer Publishing Company.

Putman, P. G., & Kriner, B. A. (2017). Using a community of practice to enhance the adjunct experience. In R. Fuller, M. K. Brown, & K. Smith (Eds.), *Adjunct faculty voices: Cultivating professional development and community at the front lines of higher education* (pp. 62-69). Sterling, VA: Stylus.

Shropshire, V. (2017). Exiting the freeway faculty path: Using professional development to get out of cruise control. In R. Fuller, M. K. Brown, & K. Smith (Eds.), *Adjunct faculty voices: Cultivating professional development and community at the front lines of higher education* (pp. 46-54). Sterling, VA: Stylus.

Smith, K., & Fuller, R. (2017). A survey of adjunct faculty developers. In R. Fuller, M. K. Brown, & K. Smith (Eds.), *Adjunct faculty voices: Cultivating professional development and community at the front lines of higher education* (pp. 73-86). Sterling, VA: Stylus.

Toth, E. (2007). Women in academia. In A. L. Deneef & C. D. Goodwin (Eds.), *The academic's handbook* (3rd ed., pp. 47-61). Durham, NC: Duke University Press.

U.S. Department of Education. (n.d.). *Family Educational Rights and Privacy Act (FERPA)*. Retrieved from https://www2.ed.gov/policy/gen/guid/fpco/ferpa/index.html

U.S. Department of Education, Office for Civil Rights. (n.d.). *Questions and answers on Title IX and sexual violence*. Retrieved from https://www2.ed.gov/about/offices/list/ocr/docs/qa-201404-title-ix.pdf

U.S. Department of Education, Office for Civil Rights. (2015). *Title IX and sex discrimination*. Retrieved from https://www2.ed.gov/about/offices/list/ocr/docs/tix_dis.html

U.S. Department of Education, Office of Planning, Evaluation and Policy Development and Office of the Under Secretary. (2016). *Advancing diversity and inclusion in higher education*. Washington, DC: Author.

U.S. Department of Health & Human Services. (2013). *Summary of the HIPAA privacy rule*. Retrieved from https://www.hhs.gov/hipaa

Weniger, G. R., & Knight, J. F. (2018). Legal matters for the health professions educator. In G. Kayingo & V. M. Hass (Eds.), *The health professions educator: A practical guide for new and established faculty* (pp. 345-358). New York, NY: Springer Publishing Company.

Whalen, S. (2012). Lessons from long-term activism: The San Francisco State University experience. In A. Kezar (Ed.), *Embracing non-tenure track faculty: Changing campuses for the new faculty majority* (pp. 146-161). New York, NY: Routledge.

White, S. E. (2018). Distance education strategies. In G. Kayingo & V. M. Hass (Eds.), *The health professions educator: A practical guide for new and established faculty* (pp. 105-117). New York, NY: Springer Publishing Company.

World Health Organization. (2010). *Framework for action on interprofessional education and collaborative practice*. Retrieved from https://www.who.int/hrh/resources/framework_action/en

Yuen, V. (2020, June 11). Mounting peril for public higher education during the coronavirus pandemic. Center for American Progress. Retrieved from https://www.americanprogress.org/issues/education-postsecondary/reports/2020/06/11/485963/mounting-peril-public-higher-education-coronavirus-pandemic

4

Understanding Institutional Types

Just as jobs in the health professions vary greatly by setting, academic positions are defined by the institutional context in which you work. In 1970, the Carnegie Classification of Institutions of Higher Education (CCIHE) developed a classification system for all accredited degree-granting colleges and universities in the United States (CCIHE, n.d.a). This classification framework is used across higher education for research purposes, and it serves as a nice resource for individuals exploring an academic career to understand institutional similarities and differences. Previously updated every 5 years, the Carnegie Classification is now updated approximately every 3 years. "The shorter cycle will better reflect the rapidly changing higher education landscape" (CCIHE, n.d.c, para. 1).

A compilation of the Carnegie Classification data in various forms is readily accessible online at http://carnegieclassifications.iu.edu. As of 2018, there were over 4300 degree-granting institutions in the United States with more than 20 million students enrolled. Gaff (2007) explained that these institutional types differ in many ways.

> They have different missions, offer different types of education, operate by different governance systems, and have different sources of financial support. They enroll different kinds of students and have different expectations for their faculties. They have quite different working conditions, professional responsibilities and salaries for faculty members. (p. 11)

The remainder of this chapter provides a very brief overview of the basic institutional types as defined by the Carnegie Classification, as well as examples of a few institutions in each category. Additionally, I briefly discuss topics, such as distance education, public vs. private funding, and for-profit vs. nonprofit institutions.

Gateley, C. A. *Clinical Practice to Academia:*
A Guide for New and Aspiring Health Professions Faculty
(pp. 45-50). © 2021 Taylor & Francis Group.

INSTITUTIONAL CLASSIFICATIONS

The Carnegie Classification categorizes institutions in several different ways. For this chapter, I focus primarily on the Basic Classification, which includes the following institutional types (CCIHE, n.d.b):

- Doctoral universities
- Master's colleges and universities
- Baccalaureate colleges
- Baccalaureate/associate's colleges
- Associate's colleges
- Special focus institutions
- Tribal colleges

Keep in mind that beyond the Basic Classification, institutions are also classified by undergraduate instructional program, graduate instructional program, enrollment profile, undergraduate profile, and size and setting. You also should remember that this classification is updated every 3 years, so an institution's classification profile may change over time. "Classifications are time-specific snapshots of institutional attributes and behavior" (Indiana University Center for Postsecondary Research, 2018, para. 3). The information in this chapter was based on the Carnegie Classifications 2018 Public Data File (Indiana University Center for Postsecondary Research, 2018). Table 4-1 provides more information about the Basic Classification and examples of each type of institution.

DISTANCE EDUCATION

A recent study by the U.S. Department of Education (2014) found that 25.8% of all students enrolled in postsecondary education were taking some or all of their coursework via online distance education. Most traditional colleges and universities now offer some type of online education coursework and, in many cases, entire degree programs. Other institutions have specialized in online education. Examples include University of Phoenix (Arizona), Capella University (Minnesota), and Ashford University (California). As with any degree program in which you are considering teaching, the most important factor to determine is whether or not the institution and the particular degree program are accredited. In other words, have they passed the scrutiny of an external accrediting body to ensure that they are providing quality education to students?

Table 4-1

Basic Classifications of Higher Education Institutions

Category	Percent of All Institutions	Degrees Granted During Update Year (Occasional Exceptions)	Additional Subcategories Based On	Examples
Doctoral universities	9.6	At least 20 research/scholarship doctoral degrees were awarded, or at least 30 professional practice degrees in 2 or more programs were awarded.	Level of research activity or focus on professional practice doctoral degrees	• University of Mississippi • Duquesne University • Belmont University
Master's colleges and universities	15.8	At least 50 master's degrees were awarded, but fewer than 20 doctoral degrees were awarded.	Overall size of program	• Bay Path University • Eastern Oregon University • Winona State University
Baccalaureate colleges	13.3	At least 50% of all degrees awarded were baccalaureate or higher, but fewer than 50 master's or 20 doctoral degrees were awarded.	Arts and sciences focus or diverse fields	• Bryn Mawr College • Athens State University • Tennessee Wesleyan University
Baccalaureate/associate's colleges	6.1	4-year colleges that awarded more than 50% of degrees at the associate's level	Associate's dominant or mixed baccalaureate/associate's	• Vermont Technical College • Alpena Community College • Pensacola State College

(continued)

TABLE 4-1 (CONTINUED)

BASIC CLASSIFICATIONS OF HIGHER EDUCATION INSTITUTIONS

CATEGORY	PERCENT OF ALL INSTITUTIONS	DEGREES GRANTED DURING UPDATE YEAR (OCCASIONAL EXCEPTIONS)	ADDITIONAL SUBCATEGORIES BASED ON	EXAMPLES
Associate's colleges	23.1	Associate's degree was the highest degree awarded.	Disciplinary focus (transfer, career and technical, or mixed) and dominant student type (traditional, nontraditional, or mixed)	• El Paso Community College • Elgin Community College • Flint Hills Technical College
Special focus institutions	31.1	High concentration of degrees awarded in a single field or set of related fields (e.g., health professions)	2-year or 4-year and area of emphasis	• LA County College of Nursing and Allied Health • St. Louis College of Health Careers • Appalachian College of Pharmacy
Tribal colleges	0.8	Members of the American Indian Higher Education Consortium	No additional subcategories	• Fort Peck Community College • Sitting Bull College • Haskell Indian Nations University

Note. Information compiled from The Carnegie Classification of Institutions of Higher Education (n.d.b) and Indiana University Center for Postsecondary Research (2018).

INSTITUTIONAL FUNDING

When exploring academic jobs, you also should consider whether an institution is public or private. There are several differences between public and private institutions, but the main difference is in their funding sources (Peterson's Staff, 2015). Public institutions receive allocations from their state legislatures and are overseen by boards of trustees who make legal and fiduciary decisions. Because state tax dollars help support operating costs, public institutions typically have lower tuition rates than private institutions. Private institutions do not receive state funding allocations and rely more heavily on funding from private donors and higher tuition rates. Beyond funding, there are other differences between public and private institutions. Public institutions are often, but not always, larger with more diverse degree offerings than private institutions. Because of the lower tuition rates, particularly for in-state residents, public institutions also tend to have a greater proportion of in-state student enrollment.

FOR-PROFIT VERSUS NONPROFIT INSTITUTIONS

Another factor you should consider when exploring academic jobs is whether the institution is a for-profit or nonprofit institution. For-profit institutions are run like a business. Owners and shareholders expect to make a profit from the service provided, in this case education. There is a high focus on providing education to as many students as possible in the most efficient manner. Tuition rates at for-profit institutions are typically higher than at nonprofits. Although financial stability is also important at nonprofit institutions, the goal is not to make a profit (Nonprofit Colleges Online, 2019). Funds received by the institution are funneled back into providing a full educational experience for students.

With this brief comparison, you may think that for-profit institutions are not a good choice for pursuing a degree or an academic job. This is not necessarily true. In both the private and public sector, there are well-run institutions that provide a great education to students. Unfortunately, there are also both public and private institutions that do not provide a quality education. You need to have a good understanding of the reputation and expectations of any institution you are considering in your job search and determine if you are a good match for that institution.

LEARNING ACTIVITIES

1. Explore the website of each higher education institution that you have attended. What information can you find about each institution regarding institutional type and funding?
2. Now go to the Carnegie Classifications website (http://carnegieclassifications. iu.edu) and see what additional information you can find out about each institution.

3. Find a list of all the accredited programs in your state or region for your specific discipline. What are the differences between the institutions?

4. Based on your understanding of the various institutional types and your individual career goals, what would be your ideal setting for a future academic position? Why?

REFERENCES

The Carnegie Classification of Institutions of Higher Education. (n.d.a). *About Carnegie classification*. Retrieved from http://carnegieclassifications.iu.edu

The Carnegie Classification of Institutions of Higher Education. (n.d.b). *Basic classification description*. Retrieved from http://carnegieclassifications.iu.edu

The Carnegie Classification of Institutions of Higher Education. (n.d.c). *News & announcements*. Retrieved from http://carnegieclassifications.iu.edu

Gaff, J. G. (2007). Faculty in the variety of American colleges and universities. In A. L. Deneef & C. D. Goodwin (Eds.) *The academic's handbook* (3rd ed., pp. 11-21). Durham, NC: Duke University Press.

Indiana University Center for Postsecondary Research. (2018). *Carnegie Classifications 2018 public data file*. Retrieved from http://carnegieclassifications.iu.edu/downloads/CCIHE2018-PublicDataFile.xlsx

Nonprofit Colleges Online. (2019). *Non profit vs. for profit colleges*. Retrieved from https://www.nonprofitcollegesonline.com/non-profit-vs-for-profit-colleges

Peterson's Staff. (2015, September 29). *Public university vs. private college*. Retrieved from https://www.petersons.com/college-search/public-university-vs-private.aspx#/sweeps-modal

U.S. Department of Education. (2014). *Enrollment in distance education courses by state: Fall 2012*. Retrieved from https://nces.ed.gov/pubs2014/2014023.pdf

5

Pursuing an Academic Position

Many people want to try out academia before deciding to make a full transition from clinical practice to higher education. The best way to gain part-time experience in an academic setting is by making contact with local educational programs in your discipline. If you do not know where to start, look at the website for your professional association. You will likely find a list of all educational programs for your profession listed by state. Although a program may not have a full-time faculty position open, many programs are continuously looking for area clinicians to help out with labs, guest lectures, and panel discussions. Send an email or letter to the program director describing your clinical experience and interest in gaining experience in academia as you explore the potential for a more permanent career transition. The remainder of this chapter is focused on helping you understand how to locate and pursue full-time academic positions in your discipline.

Before you apply for a full-time faculty position, you need to have a clear understanding about the institutional type where the professional program is located and the expectations of the type of faculty position advertised. If you have not already done so, I recommend that you start out by reviewing the various institutional types described in Chapter 4 and the differences between tenure-track and non–tenure-track positions described in Chapter 3. The expectations of faculty positions vary greatly depending on the type of educational institution. For example, a faculty position at a community college or small liberal arts institution may involve a heavy teaching load with some expectation of service on campus committees, whereas a faculty position at a large research institution may have expectations of clinical research, publication, or other scholarly activity in addition to teaching and service responsibilities. Some institutions place high emphasis on community engagement. Although your primary interest may be in teaching students, you need to understand the other expectations that come with a faculty position.

Gateley, C. A. *Clinical Practice to Academia:*
A Guide for New and Aspiring Health Professions Faculty
(pp. 51-66). © 2021 Taylor & Francis Group.

EXPLORING THE JOB MARKET FOR HEALTH PROFESSIONS FACULTY POSITIONS

There are many ways to identify faculty positions in your discipline. Some involve knowing the right people; others involve a lot more research on your part. Some academic opportunities present themselves when you are not even considering a transition out of clinical practice, whereas others may require years of patience and persistent exploration to identify a position that is the right fit for your skills and career goals.

Insider Information

One of the most common ways to learn about faculty positions is through word of mouth (Vick, Furlong, & Lurie, 2016). If you are already involved with a particular institution on an adjunct or part-time basis, you may be privy to insider information about upcoming full-time positions. If you know someone in a current faculty role who is aware of your interest in academia, he or she may notify you of an upcoming faculty position. If you are new to an area or looking to relocate, an email introduction to area program directors may result in you finding out about upcoming positions even before they are posted. See Box 5-1 for a sample email.

Institutional Websites and Professional Association Job Boards

Each institution will have a list of academic positions available with links to position descriptions and information about application procedures (Vick et al., 2016). Another great way to locate academic positions is by looking at the websites of your state and national professional associations. Many associations have some type of job listing, which may include both clinical and academic positions. Some lists may include so many positions that you will need to limit your search with keywords such as "faculty" or "instructor."

Online Searches

There are several online resources for locating academic positions. When departments or institutions are conducting a search for a faculty position, they may pay to post the position on one or more of the ever-expanding list of websites for higher education jobs. Some resources may require that you create an account to explore their job listings, whereas others allow you to search without providing any information. Keeping in mind that new resources are created each year for purposes of locating faculty positions, here is a list of some of the most common online resources at the time of this writing:

Dr. Garrard,

Good morning! My name is Jeffrey Smith, and I am a certified nuclear medicine technologist who will be relocating to your area in June of this year to be closer to family. I have accepted a part-time position at the local university hospital, and I am exploring opportunities to become involved in the education of the future generation of nuclear medicine technologists. I have reviewed your website, and I see that your program has excellent graduate outcomes in terms of graduation rate, NMTCB exam pass rate, and job placement rate.

I graduated with a BHS in Nuclear Medicine in 1994 and completed a Master of Health Administration in 2017. I have nearly 3 decades of clinical experience and 10 years of administrative experience. I also have been active in my regional Chapter of the Society of Nuclear Medicine, serving as Chapter Vice President for the past 2 years.

Please contact me should you have any need for guest lectures, lab activities, or adjunct teaching. I have always enjoyed educating nuclear medicine students in the clinical setting, and I would love to learn more about any future opportunities you may have in your academic program.

Respectfully,

Jeffrey Smith, MHA, BHS-NM, CNMT

555-555-5555

jeffreysmith@myemail.com

Box 5-1. Sample email to program director.

- HigherEdJobs (www.higheredjobs.com)
- Higher Education Recruitment Consortium (www.hercjobs.org)
- Academic Keys (www.academickeys.com)
- Inside Higher Ed (https://careers.insidehighered.com)
- HigherEd360 (www.academic360.com)
- The Chronicle of Higher Education (https://chroniclevitae.com/job_search/new)
- Indeed (www.indeed.com/q-Faculty-jobs.html)

Professional Networking Sites and Recruiting Agencies

Posting your résumé on LinkedIn or other professional networking sites is a good way for others to find you and identify you as a potential match for an academic opening. This method is typically more effective for individuals who already have some level of experience in an academic setting. There are also numerous third-party recruiting agencies, sometimes jokingly referred to as *headhunters*, that assist colleges and universities in identifying individuals for academic positions. Lundsteen (2015) cautioned that such agencies are typically looking for job candidates with more experience than individuals seeking their first academic position. Lundsteen (2015) explained the following types of recruiters:

- Retained recruiters charge their clients (academic institutions) up-front fees and then conduct searches on behalf of their clients.
- Contingency recruiters only get paid if they present the academic institution with the candidate who is hired.
- Contract recruiters are hired by institutions to screen and communicate with candidates before they begin direct communication with the institution.

"No matter the type of recruiter, please do not ever forget they are working for money—and probably won't have your best interests as a top priority" (Lundsteen, 2015, para. 5).

LEARNING ABOUT THE INSTITUTION

Once you have identified a position for which you are interested in applying, you should research information about the institution to help prepare your application materials. If you are offered an interview, you need to learn everything you can about the institution and the department before the interview.

Institutional Type and Recent Trends

As discussed in Chapter 4, there are many different types of institutions. Use the institutional website and the Carnegie Classification website (http://carnegie classifications.iu.edu) to learn about the institution's size, setting, funding, degrees offered, and student population. Find out what the recent trends are for that type of institution at the state and national level and search recent news stories about the institution. For example, is it a public research institution that relies heavily on funding from federal grants and state legislative support? Is it a technical or community college that has experienced a significant increase in enrollment and established satellite locations?

Institutional and Departmental Missions

If you have worked in a clinical setting, chances are your employer hired you based on your clinical skills and ability to contribute to the overall mission of addressing the health care needs of the individuals served by the clinical setting. Can you articulate the mission of any of the employers you have had in the past? When you are searching for an academic position, you need to be familiar with and understand the various mission statements of the department, school, campus, and/or system to which you are applying. You are no longer being evaluated on your clinical skills alone. Academic employers want to know how you can contribute to their overall missions. Referencing specific information about the institution or department in your cover letter can be the first step in convincing an employer that you are a good fit for the position, or at least worthy of an interview (Vick et al., 2016).

Potential Colleagues

In addition to becoming familiar with the mission of the department and institution to which you are applying, you should also learn about your potential colleagues to help prepare your cover letter and be ready for discussions during an interview. What kind of research, teaching, or service are they involved in? What recent publications do they have? Most departments have links on their websites that provide additional information or curriculum vitae (CV) of faculty within the department. Although you do not need to memorize every detail of their careers, be familiar enough to mention in a cover letter how your skills or interests may complement those of existing faculty. Compose a list of questions that you might ask if the interview process involves meetings or meals with faculty members from the department.

PREPARING A COVER LETTER AND CURRICULUM VITAE

Assuming that you have held some type of professional job in the past, you likely have written cover letters and résumés as part of the application process for a job. Applying for an academic job is similar, but you may need to highlight aspects of your experience beyond your clinical skills to get employers to view you as a potential candidate for an academic position. You will need to compose a cover letter that addresses the components of the job announcement and develop a CV that highlights experience that you may have relevant to an academic career.

Cover Letter

Before you begin your cover letter, carefully review the job announcement to determine the background and skills that the employer is seeking (Vick et al., 2016). You should also review information about the particular program and institution to which you are applying. Your cover letter should convey that you are qualified to meet the specific expectations described in the announcement and that you are familiar with the institution's and department's vision, history, and recent accomplishments. There are numerous online examples of how to format a cover letter.

Curriculum Vitae

Outside of academia, job seekers are often encouraged to condense their résumés into only one or two pages (Lester, 2018). A CV is typically much longer and includes experiences relevant to the academic position you are seeking (Vick et al., 2016). If you are applying for a clinical teaching position, be sure to highlight any experience you have educating students and other professionals in the clinical setting. You should also highlight any leadership, research, or service roles. Have you provided in-services or skills training to staff at your facility or in the community? Do you assist with coordinating students coming to your facility for clinicals or fieldwork? Do you serve on a departmental or facility committee focused on quality improvement? Have you assisted department leadership in writing or revising policies and procedures? Are you instrumental in new employee orientation? Have you participated in any clinical research projects? What professional associations are you involved in? Have you contributed to a newsletter, newspaper, or professional publication? Employers who are hiring someone for a clinical teaching position will not expect you to have experience in all of these areas, but they will be looking for something that makes your background stand out against that of someone with similar clinical experience. A simple online search will produce dozens of templates for formatting a CV. You may also find examples of current faculty in your discipline on their program websites. Depending on your background, your CV may include the following:

- Personal information (name, address, phone, email, and social media)
- Education
- Professional employment
- Professional activities (include scholarship, teaching, or editorial responsibilities)
- Honors and awards
- Licensure and certification
- Professional affiliations (membership and any leadership activities)
- Community involvement

SEEKING REFERENCES AND LETTERS OF RECOMMENDATION

As with any career move, you will need to recruit two or three individuals to serve as professional references for you. Some institutions will require that you submit letters of recommendations with your application, whereas others will simply ask for a list of references. In either case, you should discuss with your references your reasons for pursuing the position and why you feel qualified for the job so they know which areas to highlight in a recommendation letter or reference request. If you are transitioning from a clinical position, you may need to remind your references of experience you have that is relevant to an academic position. For example, have you supervised students during clinical or fieldwork placements? Have you provided continuing education opportunities for colleagues or community members?

YOUR ONLINE PRESENCE

You probably can think of a time when you went searching online to learn more about someone, and you formed quick opinions about that person based on the words and pictures he or she posted. Potential employers and colleagues are likely to do the same thing with you. Magness (2016) stressed the importance of leveraging your online presence to secure an academic job.

> If you are on today's academic job market, it's crucial that you have a good professional online presence. It is now possible for potential employers to Google you and look at your social media profiles. What they find could determine whether or not you get the job you're hoping for. (para. 1)

Magness (2016) suggested four things to consider related to your online presence:

1. Your name is important in your online presence. If you have a website, you want a web address that relates to your name and can be easily found. People will judge you simply based on your email address. Is an employer more likely to consider johnsmithphysicaltherapist@myemail.com or partyboy99@myemail. com as a potential candidate for a position?
2. A professional image is important in your online presence. If someone searches your name online, will they see a head shot of you or perhaps a photo with professional colleagues? Or will it be a picture of you drunk with friends at the most recent home football game?
3. Consider carefully what you say online and where you say it. Perhaps you have a blog about an area of interest or expertise related to your discipline. Beyond blogging, think about how you present yourself as a potential employee and colleague. Do you frequently complain on Facebook and Twitter about your workplace, coworkers, or life in general, or do your posts tend to focus on more positive things?
4. "Your tone compliments your content" (Magness, 2016, para. 11). Your tone includes what you choose to write about, how you say it, and where. If you are hired into an academic position, you become a representative of that institution. If your social media posts tend to be controversial or confrontational, employers may lose interest in you for a position.

SEARCH COMMITTEES

In many academic settings, a search committee consisting of a few to several individuals from the department or school will conduct the search for a new faculty member. Typically, "the search committee is formally an advisory committee to whoever has the authority to actually make the hire" (Evans, 2011, para. 2). I have served on search committees where the hiring administrator relied entirely on the search committee's recommendations. I have served on other committees where the hiring administrator made it very clear from the beginning that our opinions were important but certainly not the final say.

THE INTERVIEW PROCESS

Preliminary Interviews

Depending on the type of position for which you are applying, the institution, the number of applicants, your proximity, and a myriad of other factors, you may be asked to complete a phone or videoconference interview as a first step in the selection process. You need to be just as prepared for a digital interview as you would be for one in-person. The HireVue Team (2018) provided several recommendations for preparing for a digital interview. Although these are general recommendations applicable to all types of job searches, they are very relevant to an academic job search.

- Understand the company's culture. Learn everything you can about the institution and department before the interview and be prepared to provide answers and ask questions that demonstrate you spent time exploring this topic.
- Research who you will be working under. This person may or may not be the person conducting the digital interview, but if you make it past the initial digital interview, you likely will be interviewed by this individual during the next phase of interviews. The HireVue Team (2018) also cautions applicants to keep your digital distance. In other words, do not follow a potential boss on Twitter or request a LinkedIn connection until you have built more of a relationship.
- Know the company's product or service. For an academic position, this means knowing the student population served and the various teaching, research, and service missions of the department, school, and institution. It also means knowing something about potential competitors. If you cannot locate this information, these are good topics to ask about during the interview.
- Familiarize yourself with the company's history. Explore the departmental and institutional websites. Look for recent news stories, Tweets, and Facebook posts. This information can give you talking points for the interview, particularly in regard to how your knowledge and skills may be a good fit for the position.
- Rehearse and practice. If you have any contacts in higher education, ask them what type of questions you may encounter, and practice answering those questions. You will nearly always be asked about past success, challenges, and conflicts. Have stories prepared for these questions. Search online for "common academic job interview questions," and you will find dozens of resources. Record yourself on a computer or phone to get more comfortable in front of the camera.
- Pick the right attire. Do not make the mistake of appearing too casual in a video interview. Stick with something modest and business casual or business professional. When in doubt, always err on the side of being too formal.

- Check your technology. Be very familiar with the video platform that your employer wants you to use. Do you need to download an app? Does your computer or tablet have a good connection speed? Think about where you will complete the interview. You want to have good lighting and a quiet location. Check your video and microphone. The HireVue Team (2018) also recommends positioning the video feed near the top center of your screen so it seems like you are looking at the camera even when you are looking at the video feed on your screen.
- Decide what the opportunity to video interview means for you. Did you apply for this position just to see what would happen or are you seriously considering this position? The interviewers likely have a set list of questions to ask you. Think about the knowledge and skills that you want to highlight that may have not come across in your application.

The Campus Visit

Depending on the institution and position for which you are applying, your campus visit may consist of anything from a single 30-minute interview to an all-day event. If you are traveling from a long distance, the visit may even include meals before and after your official visit. The institution may also arrange and pay for travel costs associated with your visit. Be sure to clarify who you will be meeting with and whether there are any other expectations for the visit, such as a professional presentation. See Box 5-2 for a sample itinerary of a campus visit.

Presentation

If you are applying for an academic research position, you will likely be expected to present a brief seminar about your research. If you are applying for a teaching position or if the research position involves teaching, you may be expected to conduct a teaching demonstration. If you are expected to complete a presentation, try to find out as much information as you can about expectations.

- Is there a specific topic you should focus on? In many cases, you are given free rein to select a topic. Consider presenting on an area of expertise or a salient topic for your profession. Is there a new device or intervention that you have used in clinical practice? If you are transitioning from a clinical setting, consider preparing a presentation about what students should expect during clinical/fieldwork placements or entry-level practice.
- What, if any, technology will you have access to? Is there a computer available and a screen/projector for PowerPoint (Microsoft)? Do you need to bring your own laptop or flash drive? Will you have internet access?
- Who will be your audience, and how many people should you expect? Your audience may include faculty, students, and administrators.
- How long should the presentation be? Is it a short 15- to 20-minute presentation, or will it be an entire class period?

Dear Julia Martinez,

We look forward to meeting you during your upcoming campus visit. Here is a detailed itinerary.

Thursday, September 21

- 3:30 p.m.—Arrive to regional airport. Pick up by Angie Weston (Administrative Assistant) who will provide transportation to University Inn, approximately 30 minutes of travel.
- 5:30 p.m.—Dr. Gina Powell, Dr. Rachel Benjamin, and Dr. Bill Jamison meet you in hotel lobby to take you to dinner.

Friday, September 22

- 7:30 a.m.–8:30 a.m.—Dr. Whitney Henson, Dr. Tiffany Boswell, and Dr. Winnie Duncan meet you in hotel lobby to take you to breakfast.
- 9:00 a.m.–9:45 a.m.—Interview with Department Chair Dr. Tim Wilson
- 10:00 a.m.–10:30 a.m.—Meet with Department Faculty.
- 11:00 a.m.–11:45 a.m.—Teaching Presentation to Students and Faculty in Communication Science and Disorders Department.
- 12:00 p.m.–1:30 p.m.—Lunch at University Alumni Center.
- 1:45 p.m.–2:45 p.m.—Campus Tour with Associate Chair Dr. Lea Ann Lewis.
- 3:00 p.m.–3:30 p.m.—Meet with School of Health Professions Associate Dean Dr. Anna Booker.
- 3:30 p.m.—Dr. Brittney Swanson drives you back to airport for 6:00 p.m. return flight.

If you have questions about this itinerary, please contact Bethany Kendall (Administrative Assistant) at 555-555-5555 or bkendall@ouruniversity.edu.

Box 5-2. Sample campus visit itinerary.

If you have little or no experience with presenting in front of others, a teaching or research presentation may seem like a daunting prospect. As with any topic, you can find advice and examples online for preparing a presentation for an academic job interview. Here are a few guidelines for how to prepare for the presentation (Smith, Wenderoth, & Tyler, 2013).

- Follow instructions. If you are told to prepare a presentation for an introductory-level course of students in your discipline, prepare and carry out your presentation for students, even if your audience ends up being a small group of faculty in a simulated teaching situation. You should begin your presentation with a reminder to the audience about the intended audience of the presentation, particularly if you have included any active learning strategies that will require attendees to take on the simulated role of students. However, be prepared for reluctant participation in your planned activities.
- Do some research. Once you have determined the topic of your presentation, see if you can find information about the topic from similar courses, textbooks,

professional journals, or online resources. Does your national or state professional association have any resources that you can use? You should also explore issues related to teaching and classroom management. Does the department's web page mention a commitment to active and experiential learning? If so, they may be disappointed if you prepare a passive lecture.

- Cover an appropriate amount of material, and remember that less is more. You are being judged on how you teach the material, not how much material you can teach. Focus on only three or four major points in your presentation.
- Engage students in the classroom. Depending on when you received your initial degree in your discipline, you may have experienced some or all courses in which lecture was the primary means of instruction. As discussed in Chapters 10 and 11 of this book, institutions and students now place emphasis on active learning in the classroom. Find a way to connect with your audience and help them see why your topic is relevant to them and their future careers. Consider posing questions and asking students to break into small groups for discussions or other activities.
- Practice your presentation. In many cases, you might be applying for an academic position without your current employer's or colleagues' knowledge, but find a small group of trusted friends, family, or professional colleagues with whom to practice your presentation and active learning strategies.

Matos (2015) also emphasized the importance of an academic presentation, stating "the teaching demonstration is one of the most artificial segments of a job seeker's campus interview, yet also one of the most telling and evocative" (para. 1). Matos reiterated the importance of interacting with your audience. She offered a suggestion of bringing materials for students to make name tags so you can call on them by name throughout the presentation. Matos also encouraged applicants to avoid limiting their domain to the front of the classroom. Walk up and down the rows or aisles and engage with students. "Don't be afraid to rearrange furniture or humans (with warmth and humor, of course) to better create the physical environment that would most compliment [sic] your teaching" (Matos, 2015, para. 11). Also try to provide some context for the current class session by discussing what the audience covered in the last class period and what you will highlight in the next class. Finally, be prepared for the session to take an unpredictable path if audience members show particular interest in a point that you had not intended to spend much time on. Demonstrating flexibility within your lesson plan can be very impressive to those individuals evaluating you for this position.

Tips for Interviewing

Even if you have years of clinical experience and have aced multiple interviews over your career, interviewing for an academic position requires a different type of preparation. Your interviewers may have little doubt that you are an expert in clinical settings, but what can you bring to their department, students, and curriculum? You need to do as much homework as possible before your interview. Many departments have a description of their overall curriculum and perhaps even individual course descriptions available online. You may even be able to locate student and faculty handbooks and individual course syllabi. Learn everything you can about what and how the department teaches, and start thinking about where your knowledge and skills may fit into their curriculum (Shetty, 2007). Ask the department chair and other faculty if there are particular courses for which they are looking for coverage. However, be prepared for them to ask, "Which courses would you feel comfortable teaching?" Be honest with your responses. If you have 15 years of experience in pediatric speech-language pathology, it is fine to say that you would not be comfortable teaching a course on adult neurogenic conditions.

You may also want to explore available teaching resources, such as current textbooks, online video libraries, and clinical simulation tools. For example, do an online search for "athletic training textbooks," "respiratory therapy learning modules," "human patient simulation," or other keywords that make sense for your discipline. You do not need to be an expert on these materials, but your interviewers may be impressed if you can demonstrate that you have some knowledge about contemporary teaching practices in your discipline (Shetty, 2007). Ask questions about campus resources related to teaching. Better yet, briefly explore them on your own, and ask questions like, "I saw online that your campus has a Center for Teaching Excellence. Which of the center's professional development opportunities would you recommend a new faculty member pursue?"

Go with a list of written questions you want to ask or topics you want to highlight during discussion. Even the most experienced interviewee may go "blank" without occasionally referring to a visual checklist. If you do not already own one, purchase a padfolio where you can have your questions ready for quick reference. You can also jot down facts, thoughts, or comments that you have throughout the interview process. If you are going to be interviewing with numerous people, consider having a quick reference list of each person's position and areas of research or teaching expertise. You can discreetly check that reference list during breaks in your schedule.

One final piece of advice for your interview day: Stay off your phone! Silence it or turn it off, and only look at it when you are away from interviewers. Interviewees who are constantly looking at their cell phones give the impression that they are not 100% focused on the interview, that the interview is really not that important, or that they would rather be somewhere else (Stone & Whelan, 2018).

Negotiating Salary and Benefits

As with most topics in this book, a simple online search will result in dozens of resources that address the delicate issue of negotiating salary when pursuing a faculty position, which differs considerably from negotiating salary for a clinical position. With clinical positions, you primarily are negotiating about salary and perhaps a sign-on bonus or relocation assistance depending on the job market for your profession. With an academic position, there are many other things you should consider. Kelsky (2014) explained that "young and inexperienced [faculty] candidates simply have no idea how to interpret an offer, what to ask for, or how to ask for it" (para. 6). For example, in addition to salary and set benefits like insurance and retirement plans, academic job negotiations may include things such as start-up funds to purchase teaching materials or research equipment, computer equipment and software, lab equipment, student and staff support, office space, relocation assistance, and funds for professional development and travel expenses.

First, you have to have a general understanding of the institution and department and clear expectations of the specific position for which you have applied (Kelly, 2014; Kelsky, 2014; Randall, 2018; Zackal, 2015). Is the institution public or private? What is the funding and overall climate of the institution and department? Is it a private research institution that relies heavily on alumni endowments and grant funding from research faculty? If so, are you applying for a tenure-track research position or a non–tenure-track teaching position? Is it a public institution that has suffered years of progressive budget cuts by the state legislature? Conduct research on salaries in your discipline, in your state or region, and at the particular institution where you have been offered a job.

Randall (2018) recommended searching online salary databases by state and institution. For example, the American Association of University Professors conducts an annual nationwide salary survey. In addition to *The Annual Report on the Economic Status of the Profession* (American Association of University Professors, 2018), the information is also available via a searchable database at www.insidehighered.com. However, Kelsky (2014) cautioned against this.

> Relying on aggregate salary scales from *The Chronicle* or the American Association of University Professors for direction here will absolutely do you more harm than good, because those studies will be lumping institutions of different sizes, scales, and endowments together. Salaries are extremely local, and you must carefully calibrate your asks to the local environment. (para. 15)

If you are applying to a public institution, you should be able to locate employee salary information by using "salary database" or a similar search term along with the institution's name. Such databases are updated annually, so you can do a bit of comparative analysis from year to year to get an idea of salary increases over time for particular faculty members.

Another potential resource for information about academic salaries is your discipline's professional association (Randall, 2018). Most professional associations conduct salary surveys for their professions and provide the information in summary reports or databases. Keep in mind that such surveys will include information about clinical jobs, so you will need to search the reports or databases for information specific to academic positions. Kelsky (2014) recommends relying on personal connections you may have at the institution or within higher education.

You should also make sure you have a clear understanding of the expectations for the position (Kelsky, 2014; Randall, 2018; Zackal, 2015). Is it a 9- or 12-month position? If it is a 9-month position, will the salary be paid out over 9 months or 12 months? What are the responsibilities of the position in terms of teaching, research, and service? What are the expectations in terms of applying for promotion and tenure, if applicable? Most of these questions should have been addressed in the initial job posting and during your interview, but do not be afraid to ask clarifying questions during the negotiation process.

Once you receive an initial offer from an institution, make your list of priorities and be prepared to negotiate. Randall (2018) encouraged candidates for academic positions to think broadly about what they want in a position. What is essential vs. what would simply be nice to have? Most departments expect you to negotiate (Randall, 2018; Zackal, 2015). "Don't feel as if negotiating will start you off on the wrong foot. Not advocating on your behalf may even be perceived as a weakness" (Zackal, 2015, para. 12). However, Kelly (2014) cautions that although the old adage of "it can't hurt to ask" is true, how you ask can hurt the negotiation process. "If you make reasonable requests and are easy to negotiate with, then that is a good sign to your future colleague. However, you can destroy a relationship if you play hardball in negotiations" (Kelly, 2014, para. 1). Randall (2018) concurred, explaining that you must keep in mind that you are negotiating with your potential boss and colleague.

Kelsky (2014) explained that the initial offer will likely come by email and that you should continue to communicate via email throughout the negotiating process. "The overwhelming advantage of email is that it allows the candidate to study the offer, think about it, share it with advisors and mentors, clarify requests and priorities, and compose requests" (para. 8). Interestingly, Kelly (2014) disagreed, stating that negotiations require a personal touch that simply cannot be achieved via email. Additionally, negotiating by phone allows you to listen for cues that you might not catch via email. For example, if you start the conversation by asking if the salary is negotiable, hearing an amused chuckle and a long pause before a calculated response gives you an entirely different vibe than if the individual quickly responds with "Potentially. What salary did you have in mind?"

If you do get the impression that salary is negotiable, Zackal (2015) recommended counteroffering with a specific number, not a range. In other words, if the institution offered you a starting salary of $53,000, don't respond with "I was really hoping for somewhere between $55,000 and $60,000." Instead counteroffer with a specific number toward the top end of the range that you have researched and believe to be appropriate for the position, such as $58,000.

In some situations, salary may not be negotiable at all (Kelly, 2014). For example, small, unionized, and/or public institutions with shrinking state budget allocations may have no room to negotiate salary. Also recognize that much of the advice regarding academic salary negotiations is geared toward graduate students in research-based doctoral programs who are seeking entry-level tenure-track positions. "When it comes to non–tenure-track jobs, there is even less negotiating leverage available to job candidates than there is for tenure-track candidates. Adjunct and other fixed-term teaching positions typically are yoked to rigid, essentially non-negotiable pay rates" (Kreuter, 2012, para. 23).

LEARNING ACTIVITIES

1. Locate a list of all educational programs in your state or region. Search the websites of one or more institutions as if you intended to apply there. What did you learn about the institution? Do you have the necessary qualifications if a job became available there? Are there any recent news stories that give you more insight into current issues faced by the institution?

2. Explore the website of your state and national professional associations. What faculty jobs are listed? What are the position requirements and expectations?

3. Using one or more of the higher education job search websites listed in this chapter, search for faculty positions in your discipline. How many jobs are advertised? Are there any near you? Do you notice any trends regarding the job listings for your discipline?

4. Search for common interview questions for academic jobs. Practice answering these questions with a peer. Even better, seek out your campus Career Center and see if they offer mock interviews.

5. Explore publications specific to your discipline. Are there any articles related to faculty issues or job searches?

6. Conduct mock interviews with classmates. If possible, invite faculty or higher education administrators to conduct the mock interviews or to serve on a guest panel focused on faculty interview tips.

7. Select one faculty position advertised within your discipline, preferably at an institution in your state or another state to which you would consider relocating in the future. Learn everything you can about the institution and department.

   a. Prepare a cover letter and résumé for that position.

   b. Prepare a list of questions you would ask if you were invited for an interview.

   c. Prepare a 1-page quick reference sheet of faculty in the department along with their interests and accomplishments that you could bring up during a campus visit.

   d. Develop a list of potential topics that you could prepare for a teaching demonstration.

8. Explore online resources and develop a list of interview tips that are not covered in this chapter. If you are enrolled in a class while reading this book, work with other students to share information you located and create a master list of recommendations.

REFERENCES

American Association of University Professors. (2018). *The annual report on the economic status of the profession, 2017-2018.* Inside Higher Ed. Retrieved from http://www.insidehighered.com/aaup-compenstion-survey

Evans, D. (2011, February 28). The search committee's role. The Chronicle of Higher Education. Retrieved from https://www.chronicle.com/blogs/onhiring/the-search-committees-role/28118

HireVue Team. (2018, January 6). *Video interview preparation: 8 tips for successful video interviewing.* HireVue. Retrieved from https://www.hirevue.com/blog/how-to-prepare-for-your-hirevue-digital-interview/

Kelly, C. (2014). *It can hurt to ask.* Inside Higher Ed. Retrieved from https://www.insidehighered.com/advice/2014/03/17/essay-how-negotiate-academic-job-offers

Kelsky, K. (2014, March 24). *The professor is in: OK, let's talk about negotiating salary.* The Chronicle of Higher Education. Retrieved from https://chroniclevitae.com/news/400-the-professor-is-in-ok-let-s-talk-about-negotiating-salary

Kreuter, N. (2012, September 5). *Salary realities.* Inside Higher Ed. Retrieved from https://www.inside-highered.com/advice/2012/09/05/essay-what-new-faculty-members-need-know-about-salaries

Lester, M. C. (2018). *The one-page resume vs. the two-page resume.* Inside Higher Ed. Retrieved from https://www.insidehighered.com/advice/2012/09/05/essay-what-new-faculty-members-need-know-about-salaries

Lundsteen, N. (2015, September 14). Third-party recruiters and Ph.D. candidates. Inside Higher Ed. Retrieved from https://www.insidehighered.com/advice/2015/09/14/advice-new-phds-using-third-party-recruiters-find-jobs

Magness, P. (2016, December 21.) *4 ways to leverage your professional online presence to secure an academic job.* The Institute for Humane Studies. Retrieved from https://theihs.org/blog/professional-online-presence-academic-job

Matos, N. (2015). *Making the most of your teaching demo.* The Chronicle of Higher Education. Retrieved from https://chroniclevitae.com/news/1165-making-the-most-of-your-teaching-demo

Randall, B. K. (2018). *Academic job offer and salary negotiations.* University of Washington Graduate School. Retrieved from https://grad.uw.edu/for-students-and-post-docs/core-programs/mentoring/mentor-memos/academic-job-offer-and-salary-negotiations

Shetty, S. (2007). The job market: An overview. In A. L. Deneef & C. D. Goodwin (Eds.) *The academic's handbook* (3rd ed., pp. 136-143). Durham, NC: Duke University Press.

Smith, M. K., Wenderoth, M. O., & Tyler, M. (2013). The teaching demonstration: What faculty expect and how to prepare for this aspect of the job interview. *CBE Life Sciences Education, 12*(1), 12-18. doi:10.1187/cbe.12-09-0161

Stone, G., & Whelan, F. (2018). Ditch your cell phone and 9 other interview tips for recent graduates. Monster Retrieved from https://www.monster.com/career-advice/article/interview-tips-for-recent-graduates

Vick, J. M., Furlong, J. S., & Lurie, R. (2016). *The academic job search handbook* (5th ed.). Philadelphia, PA: University of Pennsylvania Press.

Zackal, J. (2015, July 8). *Eight tips for negotiating your salary.* Retrieved from https://www.higheredjobs.com/articles/articleDisplay.cfm?ID=700

6

Knowing Your Profession

Most health professionals enter their fields with a general understanding of their overall professions, and they gradually gain in-depth knowledge about a particular area of practice. Depending on how long you have been in practice, you may or may not have kept up on issues facing your profession beyond your immediate practice area. If you are considering an academic job, you need to have a good understanding of the major issues facing your profession at the national level, both in terms of clinical practice and educational preparation. The health care and higher education contexts are constantly evolving, and you may need to do some research on the effects of those changes on your profession. This chapter provides several recommendations of ways that you can maximize your knowledge about your profession.

STAYING CONNECTED WITH OTHER CLINICIANS

Every former and current classmate and coworker serve as a potential resource to you. Each of those individuals has a wealth of knowledge and skills that you can tap into if you obtain an academic position. College instructors in the health professions are not expected to be content experts in every specialty area of practice, but you may be expected to know who is. You may call on your professional connections months or years down the road to answer questions about their specialty areas or to be guest lecturers, panel discussion participants, clinical supervisors, or collaborative researchers. With electronic communication and social media, it is easier than ever before to maintain those connections and reach out when needed.

Gateley, C. A. *Clinical Practice to Academia: A Guide for New and Aspiring Health Professions Faculty* (pp. 67-74). © 2021 Taylor & Francis Group.

Professional Associations

It is an expectation in the academic world that you maintain membership in your state and national professional associations. Professional associations serve "to unite and inform people who work in the same occupation" and to advance practice, education, and research for their respective professions (Santiago, 2018, para. 1). Professional associations advocate for their professions in state and federal legislation that impacts practice and reimbursement. They also serve as a network of individuals who can help you advance your career and a resource for publications, continuing education, and many other services. If you have plans to pursue an academic career, you should invest in membership in your professional associations and become familiar with all the resources available to you with your membership. Beyond membership, you may be expected in an academic role to be actively engaged in your professional association by presenting at conferences or holding an officer position. If you are not familiar with the opportunities available to you, you will need to do some online exploration and talk with other academics in your discipline.

Professional association websites are a great resource for familiarizing yourself with current issues facing the profession, such as regulatory decisions, reimbursement changes, market demand for practitioners, educational trends, and emerging practice areas. Many articles and documents may be readily accessible to anyone, whereas other areas of the website may be restricted to members only. These websites may also have job listings and information about upcoming professional development opportunities.

Accreditation Standards for Health Professions Education

To become a health professional, students typically must complete an accredited degree program. What exactly does this mean? Health professions have accrediting entities, often affiliated with their national professional associations, which set the minimum educational standards that degree programs must meet as they educate students. These standards may include expectations regarding course content, qualifications of faculty and administrators, student/faculty ratio, physical space, library resources, clinical or fieldwork experiences, certification exam pass rates, and countless other aspects of education. The Institute of Medicine (2004) further described accreditation as follows:

> A voluntary process of institutional self-regulation, often conducted within the broad framework of standards established by the U.S. Department of Education and the Council for Higher Education Accreditation (CHEA). By setting standards for educational programs and methods for institutional peer review, accrediting bodies advance academic quality, ensure accountability to the public, encourage institutional progress and improvement, and provide a mechanism for continual assessment of broad educational goals for higher education. (p. 127)

As a health professions student, you probably did not know or think much about your discipline's educational accreditation standards. You likely just assumed that your professors were doing what they were supposed to do. If you pursue an academic position, you will become closely acquainted with the educational accreditation standards for your profession, particularly if your academic program is in the process of initial accreditation or accreditation renewal. Think about jobs that you have held in health care or educational settings. Was there ever a review by the Joint Commission, Department of Health and Human Services, Department of Education, or similar entity? Do you recall the level of anxiety and preparation that occurred when administrators knew that inspectors or reviewers were planning a visit? I have worked in multiple health care facilities and public schools where there was a secret code phrase that was overhead paged or texted to employees to let us know that the dreaded inspectors had actually arrived and everyone should be on their best behavior. When the on-site visit was over, most places passed inspection or accreditation, and reviewers always identified areas of strength and areas for improvement. Administrators would work quickly to address any areas of concern, educate employees about required changes in practice, and establish new methods of monitoring progress. Eventually everything would settle back down for months or years until the next anticipated inspection or accreditation visit.

Accreditation in higher education is not much different. It is an anxiety-ridden process for administrators and faculty as they strive to prove that they are doing a good job in preparing students for entry-level practice. Similar to health care settings, even though accreditation standards should be monitored and adhered to at all times, they receive the most attention when we know someone is coming to assess our performance in meeting them. If you are exploring an academic career, you will need to review your respective accreditation standards and have a clear understanding of how they impact your faculty role. You should also determine the accreditation status of any programs where you are seeking employment. You should be able to locate information about a program's accreditation status online, either on the program's website or on the accrediting agency's website. This topic is a good discussion point during interviews. Ask your potential employer the following questions:

- What are some of the biggest challenges you face in meeting accreditation standards?
- How are faculty involved in preparing for accreditation reviews and maintaining accreditation compliance?

PROFESSIONAL CERTIFICATION AND LICENSURE

As a health professions faculty member, you will need to maintain the same certification and licensure that you did as a practitioner. The educational accrediting body for your profession likely will have accreditation standards specifying this requirement. You need to be familiar with the requirements at both the national and state levels for initial and ongoing certification and licensure. Initial certification typically involves passing a national board certification for your profession. Then you must obtain professional licensure from the state in which you plan to work. Most health professions now require a minimum number of hours of continuing education or professional development to maintain or renew certification and licensure at the state and national levels.

As a clinical practitioner, you probably attended conferences related to a particular diagnosis or treatment approach. In academia, you may have the opportunity to attend conferences related to teaching, research, and other aspects of your faculty role. State and national professional association conferences are a great way to obtain several hours of continuing education at one event. You need to ensure that these types of professional development activities are recognized by the certification and licensure entities for your profession. If they are not recognized, you should develop a plan for how you will meet your continuing education requirements. This is also a topic you should bring up in interviews for faculty positions. Ask your potential employer the following:

- What opportunities exist in the department/school/campus for professional development?
- What funding is available to support faculty in attending professional development conferences at the state and national level?

PROFESSIONAL PUBLICATIONS

As discussed in Chapter 2, the term *evidence-based practice* has proliferated in the health professions in recent years. You can find dozens of explanations of evidence-based practice. Evidence-based practice can be defined as "the integration of clinical expertise, patient values, and the best research evidence into the decision making process for patient care" (Sackett, 2002, as cited in Duke University Medical Center, 2017, para. 2). If you have been in practice for several years, you may have kept up to date with research in your particular specialty area. Realistically, most practitioners are so busy with day-to-day job responsibilities and other life roles that they rarely, if ever, take time to read academic journals, textbooks, and official documents from their professional associations. However, if you are pursuing a career in academia, you need to make a priority of being up to date with professional publications in your discipline.

Official Documents of Your Profession

When you first obtained your entry-level practice degree, you were introduced to documents in your discipline that defined your profession and its purview and established guidelines for practice. When was the last time you read any of those documents? Do you even remember what they are called or where to locate them? Your national professional association website is a good place to start. The terminology varies by discipline, but try searching for "official documents," "core documents," "practice policies," "scope of practice," or "standards of practice." These documents are updated routinely and may have changed significantly since you last read them. Between the year I first obtained my entry-level degree and the time I transitioned into a full-time academic role, my profession had published the *Occupational Therapy Practice Framework: Domain and Process* (American Occupational Therapy Association, 2002), a document that did not even exist when I was a student. Now in its third edition, this is the primary document upon which our educational accreditation standards are based (American Occupational Therapy Association, 2014). Spend some time reviewing all of the official documents of your profession. You will need to be well versed in their content for interviews and in order to teach students.

State Practice Act

In addition to national practice guidelines for your profession, you also need to be familiar with your state practice act. This document defines the scope of practice for your discipline in your particular state and may be more restrictive than your national practice guidelines (American Physical Therapy Association, 2018). For example, licensed professionals may be allowed to perform particular interventions in one state but not another. In another example, some states may require that licensed professionals have a certain amount of experience before supervising students or other practitioners. You will need to have a good understanding of these differences so that you can educate students about practice issues they may encounter in their future careers.

Academic Journals

You can probably name at least one or two academic journals that publish research relevant to your profession. When was the last time you read a research article? Possibly when you last had a class assignment that required you to or maybe when you encountered a rare diagnosis in practice that you were trying to learn more about. Many health professionals simply do not make time to read academic journals or have no formalized process within their work settings to translate knowledge into practice (Kristensen, Nymann, & Konradsen, 2016). If you are pursuing an academic career, you need to familiarize yourself with current research trends. What are the "hot topics" in your profession right now? Which new treatment approaches have been developed in recent years? How do those research findings impact professional practice? Talk to individuals in academic positions to determine which journals you should peruse to get an overview of the current research in your profession. Find out how to access these journals. Do you have to be a member of your national professional association? Can you access articles through the local health sciences library? Are any research articles in your profession available through online resources, such as Google Scholar (https://scholar.google.com)?

Professional Practice Publications

In addition to academic journals that publish scholarly research, most health professions also have at least one other publication that focuses more on practice. These professional practice publications tend to include feature stories on particular areas of practice, current issues facing the profession, and new treatment approaches or equipment used in practice. They read more like a magazine or newspaper and may be available in print, online, or both. Such publications may also include job listings and advertisements for professional development opportunities. Find out which practice publications are most relevant to your discipline, and read some of the recent issues to familiarize yourself with current events in your profession.

Textbooks

As you transition to a college teaching role, one of the first things you need to determine is which textbooks you will use for your courses. If you are taking over an existing course previously taught by another professor, the textbooks may already be determined for you. However, it is a good idea to familiarize yourself with the other options that are available in your discipline. Remember how expensive textbooks were when you were a student? As a faculty member, you want to select textbooks and other resources that will be the best tools for student learning without adding tremendously to their college costs.

Once you are in an academic position, you can obtain a free copy of or electronic access to textbooks that you want to review as potential materials for your course simply by contacting the publisher. In many cases, publishers will have a salesperson assigned to your specific discipline and region. Locate this individual's contact information and introduce yourself via email or a phone call. Explain which subject areas you are teaching and ask which materials are available for review. Keep in mind that for every health professions textbook available, there is likely at least one other option available on the same subject from a competing publishing company. Shop around! Find out the leading textbook publishers for your discipline and contact all of them. In most cases, the review copies are yours to keep, even if you select a different textbook for your course. Once you get on a publisher's contact list, they may periodically send you their new publications without even having to request them. You can build quite a reference library for yourself and your students. Many textbooks also come with instructor materials, such as learning activities, sample quizzes, sample Power-Point (Microsoft) presentations, client videos, and other learning resources.

Health professions textbooks, assuming the first edition performed well on the market, are revised approximately every 5 years. Competing publishers are often looking to expand their textbook offerings, so be on the lookout for new textbooks from other publishers that cover similar material. I am always on the lookout for new materials that may enhance my students' learning. I often seek feedback from students at the end of the semester about the textbooks that I used in a particular course. Keeping in mind that students do not fully understand all that goes into planning a course, I do value their opinions about the readability and perceived usefulness of a textbook. If they found a particular textbook challenging to read and understand, perhaps there is a better resource available. On the other hand, if they found a textbook easy to read and appreciated supplemental learning materials that came with the textbook, I am likely to stick with that textbook the next time I teach the course. When new editions of textbooks come out, I carefully review them to determine if the additional cost for students is worth the new and revised material in the textbook. If you do elect to use a new edition, be prepared for students to ask you if it is okay for them to purchase an older (cheaper) edition. I get asked this question nearly every semester.

LEARNING ACTIVITIES

1. Make a list of professional contacts you have and their respective areas of expertise. Think beyond your own discipline. In health care, we work in inter-disciplinary teams, and your future students will need to understand this. Who might you call on in the future to help out with a guest lecture, panel discussion, or treatment demonstration?

2. Identify the most important professional associations that you should join. If you are unsure, reach out to colleagues in your field, particularly those in academic positions, and ask for their advice. Explore the websites of at least one state and one national professional association for your discipline.
   a. What are the annual membership dues?
   b. How many members does the organization currently have? How does that compare to the total number of practitioners in your discipline nationwide? If there appears to be a large discrepancy, what do you think are the contributing factors?
   c. What resources are available to you as a member?
   d. What are some current issues facing the profession? How is your national professional association addressing those issues?
   e. Does your professional association host an annual conference or other educational events? Have you ever attended? When is the next one? What is the cost?

3. Locate the educational accreditation standards for your profession. Are there any that were surprising to you? Is it clear how the educational program would demonstrate compliance to accreditation reviewers?

4. Pick at least one academic program in your discipline and find out the program's current accreditation status. When was the last accreditation review? When is the next accreditation review scheduled?

5. Identify at least three research journals relevant to your profession. Locate and review at least one article from each of those journals. What did you learn? How does this information impact professional practice? Set a realistic goal for yourself about routinely reviewing current evidence in your profession.

6. Identify at least one practice publication relevant to your profession. If possible, obtain a copy or access the publication online. What is included in this publication? What are some current issues facing your profession? Are there advertisements for jobs or professional development opportunities? How often is this publication produced? How long did it take you to review it? Think about when you could set aside this much time occasionally to stay up to date on current issues in your profession.

7. Go online and locate some of the leading publishing companies for your discipline. What textbooks are available for your profession? Are there similar textbooks from other publishers? Are instructor materials available?

REFERENCES

American Occupational Therapy Association. (2002). *Occupational therapy practice framework: Domain & process*. Bethesda, MD: AOTA Press.

American Occupational Therapy Association. (2014). *Occupational therapy practice framework: Domain & process* (3rd ed.). Bethesda, MD: AOTA Press.

American Physical Therapy Association. (2018). *Practice acts by state*. Retrieved from http://www.apta.org/Licensure/StatePracticeActs/

Duke University Medical Center. (2017). *What is evidence-based practice (EBP)?* Retrieved from http://guides.mclibrary.duke.edu

Institute of Medicine. (2004). *In the nation's compelling interest: Ensuring diversity in the health-care workforce*. Washington, DC: The National Academies Press. doi:10.17226/10885

Kristensen, N., Nymann, C., & Konradsen, H. (2016). Implementing research results in clinical practice: The experiences of healthcare professionals. *BMC Health Services Research, 16*(48), 1-10. doi:10.1186/s12913-016-1292-y

Santiago, A. C. (2018). *The benefits of joining professional associations*. Verywell Health. Retrieved from https://www.verywellhealth.com/professional-association-1736065

The First Year

Becoming Familiar With Your Campus, School, and Department

Think back to your first job as an entry-level practitioner in your discipline, or, if you are a student who has yet to enter your chosen profession, think back to any new job that you have had. During the job search and interview process, you learned a little bit about the organization, with emphasis on the particular department in which you would be working. Over time, you learned more about the larger organization and how your department fit into the larger mission of that organization. You gradually learned the climate and culture of your setting through formal meetings, informal conversations, and observations of what was going on around you. Chances are that a lot of what you experienced during your first year surprised you. Transitioning into an academic position can be much the same. This chapter provides an overview of how to go about becoming familiar with your campus, school, and department during your first year on the job.

UNDERSTANDING THE GOVERNANCE STRUCTURE OF YOUR INSTITUTION

State-Level Postsecondary Governance

If you have worked as a practitioner in your profession, you probably were introduced to one or two levels of administration and governance during your interview (e.g., your immediate supervisor and perhaps that individual's supervisor). During new employee orientation, you may have learned more about how your particular department fit into the overall governance structure of your particular work setting.

Gateley, C. A. *Clinical Practice to Academia: A Guide for New and Aspiring Health Professions Faculty* (pp. 75-98). © 2021 Taylor & Francis Group.

If you worked for a hospital or other health care entity, your site may have been part of a larger conglomeration of hospitals or clinics. If you worked for a public school, you knew that your school was part of a larger district, which was governed by some state-level department.

State-level postsecondary governance structures vary greatly among the 50 states. Although state-level governance may seem very far removed from your particular faculty position, it is still a good idea to have a general understanding of the governance structures in your state. The Education Commission of the States (2018) explained the following:

- "State postsecondary governance structures are critical to how state postsecondary policy is implemented and funding appropriated.
- Accountability in postsecondary education is a function of postsecondary governance.
- Issues of institutional autonomy and state control are often defined through the state governance structure.
- Governance can determine the extent that postsecondary education achieves statewide goals."

The website of the Education Commission of the States (www.ecs.org) offers individual state profiles for each state and links to comparisons of the following:

- State-level coordinating and/or governing agency
- System/institutional governing boards
- State student assistance and loan agencies
- Postsecondary vocational-technical education
- State-level organization of independent (i.e., nonprofit) colleges and universities
- Licensure/approval agencies
- Statutory advisory committee
- Additional information for each state

Institutional Governance

Institutional-level governance structures vary greatly by institutional type and size. If you are seeking employment at an institution or have recently been hired, spend some time exploring the institutional website. Can you find an organizational chart that shows where your department fits in the larger realm of the university? If you cannot locate an organizational chart, you can still gain some sense of the organization of academic departments and divisions simply by how the institution's website is organized. Following are some of the common levels of institutional governance (Carpenter-Hubin & Snover, 2013; Pye, 2007):

- Board of trustees or board of regents: The board is a group of laypersons with the responsibility to govern the institution according to its stated purposes, make decisions about institutional assets, select the chief operating officer of the institution, develop the institution, and play a role in public relations between society and the academic community. Some states have one or more systems of colleges and universities that have been grouped together, and the board may oversee the entire system rather than a single campus.

- President or chancellor: The president or chancellor of an institution is responsible for overall academic quality, public and legislative relations, and fiscal management. Depending on the type, size, and history of the institution, the president or chancellor may be involved in the recruitment and hiring of faculty or more focused on business and investment issues.
- Provost, vice chancellor, or vice president of academic affairs: This individual serves as the chief academic officer of the institution providing oversight of curriculum, instruction, academic policies, and faculty appointments and promotion. Depending on the size of the institution, this individual may also oversee student affairs, or there may be a separate leadership role for that duty, such as a vice provost or vice chancellor for student affairs. Universities that have an academic medical center may have an additional vice chancellor or vice president for the health system.
- Deans: Deans serve as administrators over a particular division or academic unit, such as a college of health professions. The responsibilities of a dean may include handling a variety of faculty, staff, and student issues as well as strategic planning and advocacy for the academic unit, accreditation and program review, and economic development. Large academic divisions may also have one or more associate deans.
- Department chairs: Department chairs serve as the business managers and academic leaders for their departments. They are accountable for allocating resources to support the mission of the department while ensuring that the department's business practices conform to institutional rules. Unlike the other administrators described earlier, department chairs remain members of the faculty with expectations for teaching and/or research in addition to their administrative responsibilities. Depending on the size and complexity of a department, individual academic units may have separate program directors who assist department chairs with management and leadership of specific programs.

Shared Governance

In 1920, the American Association of University Professors (AAUP) issued a statement on the subject of shared governance, "emphasizing the importance of faculty involvement in personnel decisions, selection of administrators, preparation of the budget, and determination of educational policies" (AAUP, n.d.b, para. 2). After numerous refinements, the *Statement on Government of Colleges and Universities* (AAUP, 1966) was jointly released by the AAUP, the American Council on Education, and the Association of Governing Boards of Universities and Colleges. The statement calls for cooperation and shared responsibility among the various components of academic institutions in matters of internal operations and educational policy, including curriculum oversight and determination of faculty status. Each institution will have a different interpretation and operationalization of shared governance. "Powers of faculty bodies are normally the product of a long history of negotiation between faculty and administrators and boards" (Pye, 2007, p. 357).

Following are just a few examples of shared governance that you may encounter (Kezar, 2012; Melear, 2013; Pye, 2007):

- Faculty senate: A faculty senate is a representative body of faculty that serves as a forum for debating educational policy issues relevant to divisions across the institution. Faculty senate composition and purview vary by institutional type and history. For example, at some institutions, only tenured and tenure-track faculty are represented on the faculty senate. On unionized campuses, the faculty senate may focus on academic concerns, whereas the faculty union focuses on employee salaries and benefits.

- Curriculum committee: Curriculum committees may exist at the department, school, and campus levels. Their purpose is to provide oversight and approval of new course offerings, course changes, and course discontinuances.

- Policy committee: Policy committees typically exist at the school and/or campus level. Their purpose is to develop and review proposed policies, ensuring that each policy is consistent with the mission and priorities of the institution and in alignment with campus- or system-level regulations.

There are numerous other types of standing committees, ad hoc committees, and task forces that exist on campuses. Standing committees are permanent committees with responsibilities of conducting ongoing work. Ad hoc committees are created for short-term purposes to address a particular issue or goal. I recommend that you explore whether shared governance exists on your campus and, if so, to what extent. Talk with colleagues. Explore institutional websites. Find out from your department chair which committees exist at the department, school, and campus level. Where might you be asked to serve within your first few years in a faculty position? Pye (2007) warned against getting too involved in faculty governance issues early in an academic career, particularly for individuals on the tenure-track where research productivity may be the primary factor impacting tenure decisions.

> Young professors who participate in governance extensively may do so at their own peril. If they can do so without prejudice to their research, it will not be held against them. But every minute diverted from research is time not devoted to achievement of the primary requirement for advancement. (pp. 364-365)

In my own experience as a non–tenure-track faculty member, I have learned much about how my university functions from participating on committees and task forces at the department, school, and campus levels. Just like any other part of your job, if you go into committee work with a negative attitude, you will likely hate every minute of it. Instead, if you view it as an opportunity to learn, grow, network, and affect change, your experience will be much better.

BRIEF OVERVIEW OF ORGANIZATIONAL THEORY

If you are interested in pursuing a career in academia, it is helpful to have at least a general understanding of organizational theory as it relates to higher education. "Trustees, parents, and external stakeholders are frequently perplexed by characteristics of higher education organization that are absent in other organizations such as corporations, political institutions, or other nonprofits" (Manning, 2013, p. 8). These characteristics include the following:

- Highly professional employees: Faculty are experts in their field, giving them professional authority. Administrators also have advanced degrees and expert knowledge.
- Presence of cosmopolitans: Faculty have loyalties that extend beyond their current institution, such as to their alma maters and discipline-specific professional associations.
- Multiple organizational structures: "Several organizational structures occur simultaneously within colleges and universities.... Few other organizations have the complexity resulting from these simultaneously occurring structures" (Manning, 2013, p. 8).
- Conflict over the appropriate product of higher education: Although an educated person may be the true product of higher education, college and university performance is often measured in terms of credit hours, graduation and retention rates, and faculty productivity in teaching and research.
- Multiple, often-conflicting roles: "Faculty, administrators, staff, students, and external stakeholders by structure, temperament, and responsibilities play vastly different roles within higher education organizations" (Manning, 2013, p. 8). The roles of these individuals are often at odds with each other, further complicating organizational structures within higher education.

There are entire textbooks and graduate-level courses dedicated to this topic if you have interest in gaining a more in-depth understanding of organizational theory to analyze how a particular institution, or part of an institution, operates. Assuming that most readers of this book need only a basic overview at this point in your careers, let me briefly summarize for you some of the key literature on this topic. Over 3 decades ago, Birnbaum (1988) published a book called *How Colleges Work: The Cyberkinetics of Academic Organization and Leadership*. Birnbaum explained four organizational models of academic leadership that may be observed at various levels of an institution:

1. Collegial model: In this model, the viewpoints of all members are valued, and major decisions are made by the group as a whole. Although this model encourages group discourse and shared power, major decisions are often difficult to make because no single entity has authority.

2. Bureaucratic model: In this administrative model, organizations are divided into hierarchical levels and departments with distinct purposes and clearly defined job descriptions intended to increase efficiency. This model allows for more decisive leadership, but there may be confusing overlaps of authority within organizational layers.

3. Political model: Similar to the bureaucratic model, institutions using a political model are divided into smaller units, but groups typically have different goals and are competing for power and resources. This model emphasizes the relationships and coalitions between leaders within the institution.

4. Anarchical model: Institutions using an anarchical model lack central authority, and individuals within the organization have greater autonomy. Decisions can be made quickly, but because there is limited oversight, goals of one department may conflict or overlap with goals from another department, thus creating inefficient use of resources.

Recognizing that much has changed over the last 3 decades in regard to higher education and the challenges facing society in general, Manning (2013) claimed that "the tried and true frames so familiar in the past are currently inadequate to the task of getting out ahead of the changes that are occurring and that show no signs of abating" (p. xii). With this in mind, she expanded the discussion on organizational theory in higher education by summarizing the following four models:

1. Cultural model: The cultural model as applied to higher education relies on such things as history, ritual, tradition, and legacy in making decisions that will impact the institution's future. However, this administrative model is not always in alignment with contemporary issues in higher education such as globalization, affordability, and economic priorities.

2. New science model: The new science model provides an understanding of higher education institutions as highly interconnected with their environments. In this model, colleges and university structures are viewed as "heterarchical structures that cooperatively network in a loose state and federal structure.… The goals of each structure combine to form a regional, federal, and global system that offers higher learning, enacts social changes, enables class mobility, and realizes social justice" (Manning, 2013, p. 142).

3. Feminist model: The feminist model views colleges and universities as organizations that create, reflect, and reinforce gender dynamics within society. "Charged with the transmission of cultural knowledge, colleges and universities are collectively a major social institution that creates and sustains gender differences" via "topics covered in the curriculum, symbols and images portrayed on campus, and routine work practices where gender is explicit although often unexamined" (Manning, 2013, p. 160).

4. Spiritual model: The spiritual model, as applied to organizational culture in higher education, focuses on each individual's journey for meaning and interconnectedness. "Although people pursue higher education for many reasons, including materially driven purposes, students, faculty, and administrators are fundamentally and developmentally changed through their campus experiences.

The purposes of higher education encompass the fulfillment of human potential, social justice, and social change" (Manning, 2013, p. 185). Although this model provides a positive view of institutional organization, it may be viewed as overly optimistic and insufficient in analyzing academic leadership.

Each of the models briefly summarized earlier can be used to help understand how colleges and universities function as complex organizations. These concepts will begin to make more sense as you are immersed into your own institution as a new faculty member. Although they are not often articulated by administrators, you will begin to see examples from one or more of these models in play as you think about how and why decisions are made at the department, school, and campus levels.

LEARNING CAMPUS CLIMATE AND CULTURE

"It is absolutely necessary to familiarize yourself with the climate and culture of your new institution and department.... This should be an ongoing process, both prior and subsequent to accepting a position" (Moe & Murphy, 2011, pp. 63-64). Underlying values and beliefs constitute an institution's culture, whereas institutional climate is established through the attitudes and behaviors of the individuals at the institution (Peterson & Spencer, 1990). Although you should gather as much information as possible about the institution before interviewing and accepting a faculty position, you may not get a true sense of the climate and culture of an institution until you are immersed in it. You will gain a lot of information through informal observations and interactions, but there are also several specific resources and events that can help you learn more about your institution's climate and culture.

Mission Statements

Explore the mission statements of your institution or campus system. Depending on the size and type of institution, you may also be able to locate mission statements at a division and department level. The mission statement can tell you a lot about an institution's values and priorities. For example, suppose you have accepted a faculty position in one of the health sciences programs at Moraine Valley Community College in Illinois.

> The mission of our college is to educate the whole person in a learning-centered environment, recognizing our responsibilities to one another, to our community, and to the world we share. We value excellence in teaching, learning and service as we maintain sensitivity to our role in a global, multicultural community. We are committed to continuous improvement and dedicated to providing accessible, affordable, and diverse learning opportunities and environments. (Moraine Valley Community College, 2018, para. 1)

Based on what you learned about various institutional types in Chapter 4, it should come as no surprise that this community college is focused on teaching, learning, and service to the community. Now let's take a look at the mission statement from a different type of institution.

> The mission of the University of Missouri System, as a land-grant university and Missouri's only public research and doctoral-level institution, is to discover, disseminate, preserve, and apply knowledge. The university promotes learning by its students and lifelong learning by Missouri's citizens, fosters innovation to support economic development, and advances the health, cultural, and social interests of the people of Missouri, the nation, and the world. (University of Missouri, 2018, para. 1)

This statement also includes learning as one part of the mission but note the emphasis in the first sentence on research activity, which is characteristic of doctoral-level institutions.

Strategic Plans

In addition to mission statements, you should also take time to review institutional, divisional, and departmental strategic plans. Just as any business must periodically make adjustments to remain successful in an ever-changing environment, institutions of higher education also engage in a strategic planning process. Although changes in administration may trigger new strategic planning initiatives, typically colleges and universities take on the revision of strategic plans approximately every 5 years. Hassanein (2017) identified five common steps to the strategic planning process:

1. Selecting a strategic planning steering committee
2. Formulating or revising institutional mission and vision statements
3. Conducting a scan of both the internal and external environments to identify strengths, weaknesses, opportunities, and threats
4. Identifying key performance indicators and setting benchmarks
5. Setting specific strategic goals and related action plans

Individuals seeking to transition from clinical practice to academia are not typically thinking about the strategic plan of an institution, but strategic planning priorities can influence the climate and culture of an institution. You should be able to locate your institution's strategic plan with a simple online search.

Faculty Unions

Unionization of higher education faculty dates back to the early 1900s. Early faculty unions were focused on improving financial support for institutions and protecting academic freedoms, but they did not yet have the powers of collective bargaining that came with the unionization movement of the 1960s and 1970s (HigherEdJobs, 2012). Dr. Timothy Reese Cain, in an interview for a HigherEdJobs article (2012), explained that faculty may have many reasons for joining a union including "salary, working conditions, faculty governance, and procedural protections for academic freedom and tenure" (para. 8). However, although many view unions as a way to improve communication between faculty and administrators, others view unions as a threat to collegiality (AAUP, 2010). The AAUP views unions as an effective way for faculty and other academic professionals "to ensure their professional standing and protect themselves from the threats and challenges presented by the corporatization of American colleges and universities" (AAUP, n.d.a, para. 4).

If you are exploring a faculty position, find out if a faculty union exists for your institution. If so, explore the union website, union documents, and recent news stories to see which issues have been the focus of union activities at the institution. At some institutions, faculty unionization has long been the norm, whereas at other institutions faculty unionization may be a new and controversial topic. Consider asking a few very broad questions during the interview process, such as, "While doing some online research about the institution, I discovered that there is a faculty union on this campus. Can you tell me more about that?"

Faculty Meetings

Your department likely will have weekly or monthly faculty meetings to bring faculty together to discuss relevant issues and to disperse information from your department chair and higher-level administrators. Whether or not your attendance at such meetings is considered mandatory, you should make every effort to attend on a regular basis. Thinking back to my first year as a faculty member, these weekly department meetings were where I learned the most about my colleagues, my department, and my institution.

Your institution may also have faculty meetings at the division or campus level, typically only once or twice per semester. Again, these are great forums for learning more about your institution. It also helps you make connections with other faculty and administrators with whom you would otherwise have little contact. I remember during my first year being told by a more seasoned colleague, "Oh, you don't really have to go those school and campus faculty meetings if you don't have time." I went anyway, just to soak up as much information as I could, and I was glad I did. After attending three or four school-level meetings, and often being the only faculty member in attendance from my department, the dean of our school, who I had no idea at the time even knew who I was, said to me, "I'm glad to see that you always attend these meetings. I notice those things. It's important that someone be here to represent your department." His comments made a huge impression on me as a novice faculty member. Not only was I gaining valuable information and networking with colleagues, I was also representing my department and gaining a reputation within the school. Admittedly, I do not make it to as many campus-level faculty meetings as I should, but when I have attended, it has been a great opportunity to gain a better understanding of campus climate and culture.

Other Campus Events

Your campus will have countless other events to which faculty receive invitations, ranging from expert lectures of visiting scholars to inauguration events of new campus administrators. You will learn about such events through emails and electronic calendar invitations. You will not have time to attend everything but make time to attend a few events each semester. Each semester I try to attend one event that interests me and one event that may benefit my department or me simply through my presence and networking. For example, I once attended a presentation by Marlee Matlin, an American actress who spoke about deaf culture and perceptions of disability, topics of interest to me as a health care professional. Another time, I attended a holiday open house at the chancellor's residence on campus. I initially felt way out of my league as a new faculty member, but the chancellor was very welcoming and asked me about the successes and challenges in my department that he should know about. I also met faculty from all over campus, which added to my list of familiar faces at future campus events.

Organize and Read Your Email

When I worked in a clinical setting, I had a work email address that received a few emails per day from hospital administrators. I also used that email address for coordinating student clinical rotations with multiple academic institutions. Because I was busy with clinical care, I checked that email once daily, at best. When I started my full-time faculty position, I was surprised at the volume of daily emails I received. In addition to emails that were directed to me individually, I received emails and daily or weekly newsletters from my school of health professions, the campus, and our academic health care system. Over the years, I went from receiving perhaps a dozen emails per day to sometimes receiving 100 or more emails per day. I learned to manage my in-box by creating different folders, so I can quickly scan and prioritize which emails need my attention first, if at all. For example, I set rules where emails from particular senders get filtered to a folder called "Campus Updates." I have another folder that contains only emails from my department chair. If I check my email and have 20 new emails, I know that emails from him are likely more pressing than the weekly update about various campus events. Although it may be the last email I look at, I still skim through the weekly campus update to see if there are any events or professional development opportunities that pertain to my role and interests.

Weekly and monthly email updates from campus administrators also provide a lot of information about campus climate and culture. In recent years, my campus received a lot of national media attention for campus events surrounding racial tensions. In subsequent years, our campus saw declining enrollments, decreased state funding, and hiring freezes. Although most of our health professions programs maintained enrollment, we all felt the budget cuts and the shift in overall campus climate. The periodic email updates provided information about how administrators were responding to those issues. We now have new leadership at the campus and system level, enrollment is trending upward again, and our email updates from administrators focus more on positive stories about faculty, staff, and students.

CAMPUS RESOURCES

Faculty Handbooks or Policy Manuals

You may have faculty handbooks or policy manuals available at the department and/or school level. I had no idea such things existed when I began in my faculty role. Although they serve mainly as a resource for faculty, consulted only occasionally for particular situations, faculty handbooks and policy manuals likely contain information that will eventually be of interest to you. For example, my school of health professions has a faculty policy manual that explains administrative, academic, and promotion and tenure policies. If I have a student in danger of academic probation, I need to consult that manual to ensure that I am following school policies about how to handle the situation. That policy manual also explains in detail the various faculty ranks (e.g., clinical instructor, assistant clinical professor, associate clinical professor, clinical professor) and the process for applying for promotion from one level to the next.

If you are not introduced to these resources when you begin your faculty position, go looking for them. They are likely available in your school or department or posted on their websites. Although you may not need them initially, it is a good idea to at least skim the contents so you know what information is contained in them that you might refer to at a later date.

Campus Rules and Regulations

In addition to your department- and school-level policies, your institution will have campus- or system-level rules and regulations that pertain to all academic divisions. Policies at the department and school level must align with campus and system rules and regulations. You should be able to locate your campus rules and regulations online. Like the department- and school-level manuals, it is a good idea to at least skim the table of contents of the campus- or system-level rules and regulations so that you are familiar with regulations that may affect you as a faculty member. For example, my institution's rules and regulations specify exactly how I must handle suspected violations of academic integrity by students. Whether or not the student and I come to an agreement about my class-level sanction, I am required to report the incident to the provost's office. If it is the student's first incident of academic dishonesty, the provost's office likely will take no further action. However, if the student has had two or more allegations of academic dishonesty or if the incident is considered a particularly egregious violation, the provost's office may impose additional sanctions up to suspension or expulsion from the university. As you can well imagine, such situations are not pleasant for anyone involved, but you need to know and abide by the rules set forth by your institution.

Disability Center

Regardless of the institutional type or degree program, chances are that you will encounter students who have disability accommodations. Recent government figures indicate that about 11% of undergraduate students have a disability ranging from dyslexia and attention-deficit/hyperactivity disorder to orthopedic, vision, and hearing impairments (National Council on Disability, 2015). As more students have Individualized Education Programs and 504 plans for accommodations at the pre-K–12 level, colleges are also seeing a rise in students needing accommodations to be successful in the higher education setting. Accommodation needs are determined on an individual basis and may include any of the following:

- Adaptive equipment
- Alternative formats
- Personal assistants for reading or classroom/lab participation
- Interpreters
- Note-taking assistance
- Exam accommodations (often in the form of extended time and reduced distraction environments)
- Flexible attendance

At the pre-K level, schools have the responsibility for making sure all relevant individuals know about a student's accommodations and how to meet them. At the college level, students are responsible for working with the disability center to determine necessary accommodations and to notify each individual instructor of the accommodations needed for each course. I encourage you to become familiar with the disability center and reach out to the staff there when you have questions about how best to serve a student's needs while maintaining the learning expectations of your course. I also recommend meeting with each student on an individual basis to discuss the accommodations and how they will be addressed in your particular course. For example, if a student needs extra time and a private space to take the exam, will you be providing that time and space for the student within your department? Or will you be sending the exam to the disability center and expecting the student to handle scheduling arrangements on his or her own? Be sure to check with colleagues to see what the department's policies and expectations are for handling these situations. Within my own department, we typically can arrange a time and place for one student to take an exam with extended time and reduced distraction, but we simply do not have the space and staff to proctor exams when we have multiple students in the same class that need accommodations. In those instances, we send the exam to the disability center and have students make arrangements to take the exam at the center.

Academic Success Center

Nearly every contemporary higher education institution has some form of an academic success center or student success center that provides services, such as introducing effective study strategies, tutoring, and writing review services. If you have students who are struggling with basic skills essential for success in your course, you should try to connect them to these resources. Students may not know these resources exist or may be embarrassed to seek out academic support services. However, over my decade of full-time college teaching, I have witnessed a precipitous decline in students' basic writing skills, which impacts their performance in professional-level coursework in which they are expected to produce scholarly writing and accurate clinical documentation. I have also witnessed students struggle with the transition from prerequisite coursework into professional programs with a significant increase in academic rigor. Students are never too old to learn new study and organizational strategies. You may even consider introducing these campus resources at the beginning of the semester or including them as part of a program orientation.

Career Center

At some institutions, career exploration and preparation services may be part of the student success center. Other institutions may have a separate center focused specifically on services such as administration and interpretation of career interest and personal strengths surveys, résumé preparation, mock interviews, internship exploration, and hosting career fairs. At larger institutions, you may find career centers at the divisional level, such as within a school of health professions. As with other campus resources, you should learn about the services offered and think about how you can connect students to these resources. For example, you may design an assignment that requires students to explore a job opportunity, prepare a cover letter and résumé, and make an appointment with the career center to participate in a mock interview.

Counseling Center

I had no idea when I began college teaching how big of a role I would play in connecting students to campus mental health services. I will discuss the rising incidence of mental health issues among college students more in Chapter 9. In addition to their academic responsibilities, most students are juggling part-time employment and numerous other life commitments, leading to high levels of stress and anxiety. Even for students who find a good balance, sometimes life presents challenges that make it difficult for students to focus on academics. Grandparents have strokes or get cancer. Friends die in tragic accidents. Parents get divorced. Serious relationships fall apart. Students are shunned by family when then announce they are part of the lesbian, gay, bisexual, transgender, and queer (LGBTQ) community. When these things happen, you unexpectedly may end up with a student sobbing in your office. Of course, you should provide some level of emotional support when appropriate, but you also need to know your boundaries as an instructor or academic advisor and recognize when to refer a student to professional counseling services available on your campus. It has been my experience that students are reluctant to seek services out on their own. On several occasions, I have made a call to the counseling center on my campus, explained that I had a student in emotional crisis, and accompanied the student to the center to get connected with the appropriate professional services. Speaking from personal experience, I recommend you find the number for your campus counseling center and keep it in a handy location for quick access so you are not scrambling to look it up when you actually need it in a crisis situation.

International Center

Depending on the size and type of institution where you work, your campus may have an international center that serves as a resource for faculty, staff, and students. This office may assist international students in maintaining compliance with federal immigration regulations. It may also serve as a resource for connecting students to other individuals from their home country on the campus and in the community. Additionally, an international center may host or facilitate campus events that celebrate various cultures. These events are an excellent experience for students entering the health professions who will be encountering diverse client populations in their future careers. On a larger scale, you may be able to collaborate with staff from the international center to arrange a study-abroad experience relevant for your health professions students.

Center for Teaching Excellence

Many institutions have established a center for teaching excellence to provide teaching support, resources, and professional development opportunities for faculty across campus. In some cases, this center may have a physical location. In other cases, it may exist as an online entity. In either case, centers for teaching excellence serve as excellent resources for new and experienced faculty who want to improve their teaching. If such a center does not exist on your campus, simply do an online search for centers at other institutions. You will find numerous free resources that may be helpful to you.

Library Resources

Familiarize yourself with the library resources available on your campus. Depending on how long ago you attended college, you may have spent hours in the library studying and searching for books and articles related to your coursework, or you may have never set foot inside your campus library. Today's college students rely heavily on online search tools to gather information. However, they may be relying on Google and Wikipedia as their primary sources. If they are entering a health professions program, they may have no idea how to conduct a search for scholarly peer-reviewed articles through a discipline-specific database. Find out which resources are available to you and your students. Your campus may have a librarian or even an entire library specific to the health professions. There may be online trainings that you can use in your courses, or you may be able to have a librarian come to your class to conduct a demonstration. Even better, set up a scavenger hunt activity for students at the library so they can familiarize themselves with the resources available to them. The library system on my campus has a plagiarism module and quiz that I incorporate into first semester courses to help students better understand what constitutes plagiarism and the consequences they will face if they engage in academic dishonesty.

Technology Resources

Technology is so integrated into our daily lives that we rarely give thought to it until it does not work and causes us an inconvenience. I certainly have experienced my share of technology crises in my academic role, including forgotten passwords, locked-up learning management systems, rampantly spreading Trojan viruses, and computers that are not communicating with printers when I need to print something *now*; the list goes on and on. Know who to call when things go wrong. Is there an information technology (IT) department on your campus or a point person for your department or school? IT departments often provide trainings for tools that you may use in your academic role. For example, I had been in clinical practice for years with limited need to keep up with products such as Microsoft Outlook, Word, Excel, and PowerPoint and Adobe Acrobat. When I began my faculty role, I attended several trainings through our campus IT division to bring myself up to date with technology relevant to my new academic role.

Depending on the size of your campus, there may be a separate office or center that handles educational technology, such as learning management systems like Canvas, (Instructure Inc.) Blackboard, and Moodle. These learning platforms allow you to create a site for each course through which you can post syllabi and assignments, communicate with students, allow online assignment submissions, administer online quizzes, and enter grades. Your campus may offer trainings for faculty who are new to the campus and for existing faculty who are seeking to advance their educational technology skills. My campus occasionally offers grants and other incentives to encourage faculty to integrate technology into their teaching. Find out what resources and support are available to you.

Other Campus Resources

Every campus will have its own combination of student and faculty support services. Explore your institution's website, and talk to colleagues about resources that you should know about for your students and yourself. Although not an all-inclusive list, you may find that your campus has a Black cultural center, an LGBTQ center, a women's center, a family resource center, a veterans center, a wellness center, and countless other resources that may be helpful to you or your students.

Understanding Promotion and Tenure Guidelines

Early in your new faculty role, you need to learn about the rules for promotion and tenure at your institution (Project Kaleidoscope, 2009). I was so excited to accept my first full-time faculty position that the potential for promotion in the future never even crossed my mind. Coming from years of clinical practice, I was not even aware when I was hired that there were specific policies and procedures for promotion and tenure for faculty members. A few years after I began teaching at the college level, one of my department colleagues was promoted from assistant clinical professor to associate clinical professor. That was the first time I recall becoming aware that promotion was something I should be thinking about. My department was in a time of transition at that point with an ongoing search for a new department chair. I asked a few questions of other department faculty and learned that there was something called a *dossier* that I would need to put together to be considered for promotion, but that I could not submit the dossier until I had been in my current position for at least 4 or 5 years. I got the impression that I would receive more guidance when the time came.

A former colleague became our interim department chair and was later appointed to the permanent position. She encouraged me to consider going up for promotion. I learned that the guidelines for the promotion of non–tenure-track faculty were outlined in our school-level faculty policy manual, a document I had occasionally heard about during school-wide faculty meetings but never had actually explored. Additionally, I had to review promotion documents published by the provost's office, many of which were written specifically for tenure-track faculty with an emphasis on research publications, and try to figure out which criteria applied to me. I found the entire process confusing and frustrating, and, at the time, there were few supports in place at the school and campus levels to guide non–tenure-track faculty through the promotion process.

In retrospect, I should have learned about the promotion guidelines much earlier in my academic career. It would have made compiling the dossier much easier. As it turned out, I spent a few months trying to locate information and explain everything I had accomplished over the past 5 years. For example, I had to gather course evaluation scores and student comments from every course I had ever taught along with the department averages from each semester for comparison. I had to write a statement of my teaching philosophy. I had to have peer reviews of my teaching, which included classroom observations and review of my course materials. I had to explain my service and scholarship contributions and how they related to the documented workload distributions for my position, which had changed since I was originally hired.

I also learned that the promotion process is a long, drawn-out affair. I submitted my first promotion dossier in late summer 2013, and it went to a committee on review (COR) at the department level. After a few months, I received feedback and was required to make some modifications to the dossier, which then moved forward to my department chair. She wrote a letter of support and forwarded the dossier to a school-level COR. Over the next few months, the school-level COR provided additional feedback, and I again made modifications to the dossier. Next, the dossier was reviewed by the dean of the school of health professions, who wrote an additional letter of support and forwarded the dossier to the provost's office for final review. In spring 2014, I received official notification that I successfully had been promoted from assistant teaching professor to associate teaching professor, with an official title change and a small bump in salary effective in September 2014, nearly 18 months after I began compiling the dossier.

I am currently in the midst of my second application for promotion, this time from associate teaching professor to teaching professor. I swore to myself after my first promotion process that I would do a better job of keeping track of the things I needed for the next dossier, and then life happened. I was busy with work, family, earning a PhD, presenting at conferences, being involved in my national professional association, revising a book, writing a new book manuscript, and a dozen other commitments. I did manage to keep a running list of activities to include in the promotion dossier, but I still ended up spending a few months gathering everything I needed to compile the dossier for submission in summer 2018. I also had a better understanding this time of the overall promotion process, having served on a school-level policy committee, a school-level promotion committee for non–tenure-track faculty, and a campus-wide task force aimed at streamlining promotion policies and procedures across all divisions of the campus. My school and campus have made significant improvements to supporting non–tenure-track faculty in the promotion process over the past several years. However, even with all my insider knowledge and the additional supports, submitting a dossier for promotion was still a daunting and time-consuming process.

In summary, if you are not introduced to promotion guidelines when you are hired into a faculty position, start asking questions and learn as much as you can about the process within your first year. "It is important that new faculty investigate and understand both the policies and the implicit definitions of performance evaluation with their institution" (Brock & Symington, 2018, p. 263). Each campus will have different promotion guidelines, and those guidelines may differ between divisions. The process for promotion within your college of health professions may be different than it is in the college of business or the college of engineering. It is never too early to start preparing for promotion, even if it may be years away and not high on your priority list at the moment. Knowing what the expectations are for promotion will help you make informed decisions about which opportunities for service, leadership, scholarship, and professional development you should pursue. For example, at a recent department meeting, our department chair explained the need for someone in our department to serve on a new school-level committee. A junior faculty colleague said, "That will probably look good later on my CV [curriculum vitae] for promotion. I'll do it."

ESTABLISHING RELATIONSHIPS

It may seem like common sense, but you need to put effort into establishing good relationships with people in your new work environment when you begin a new faculty role. Unlike a new clinical position in which there likely is a structured orientation process for new employees, new faculty members may find themselves sitting in their offices wondering, "Well, now what do I do?" after the human resources paperwork and initial introductions are completed on the first day. Even though your new colleagues probably are excited to have you there, they are busy with their own research agendas, course preparation, service on committees, and all the other department work that you will eventually learn about. Unless they have been tasked with a specific part of your orientation process, you may get an occasional "Hey, how are things going?" inquiry, but other than that, it is just business as usual for them. I definitely remember feeling a little lost during my first few weeks as a new faculty member. I did not know what to ask, and I did not know who to ask. Moe and Murphy (2011) explained this phenomenon well.

> Matters of most immediate and pragmatic concern to new faculty (i.e., parking, office equipment, book orders, class rosters, audiovisual needs) are often informally contingent on the availability and helpfulness of department staff. Meanwhile, matters of greatest salience to a new faculty's future (standards of retention, tenure, and/or promotion) are often relegated to ambiguously written statements and conversations with department chairs and more senior colleagues. Given that different people may have distinct interpretations and perspectives on these standards, new faculty sometimes feel as though their coworkers are either apathetic, lack collegiality, or are even outright antagonistic. (p. 59)

My advice to you is to spend any spare time you have during your first year building relationships with your new colleagues. Keep in mind, of course, that they are all very busy people, but ask if they have time to meet briefly with you so you can learn more about their roles and how you will be working with them in the future. The following sections contain topics and questions you may want to cover during formal and informal conversations.

Department Chair

You likely spent time with the department chair during your interview process, but how much do you understand about that person's roles and responsibilities? In addition to any teaching and research obligations, the department chair also may be responsible for faculty and student recruitment, hiring and firing, faculty and staff development, budgeting, strategic planning, accreditation, fundraising, alumni relations, and numerous other aspects of department management and leadership (Buller, 2012; Colton, 2007). Ask if your department chair has time for a brief meeting to discuss his or her responsibilities. If not already discussed, use this meeting as a time to clarify expectations that the department chair has for you in terms of teaching, service, and scholarly productivity. When are performance reviews conducted? Which factors are considered in performance reviews? What are key goals the department chair has for the department over the next few years? What might your role be in helping the department achieve those goals?

Faculty

You probably already know a little about your department colleagues from the interview process. Depending on the size of your new department, I recommend trying to have at least a brief conversation with each faculty member about their current roles. "Most academics love an opportunity to talk about themselves and their work" (Moe & Murphy, 2011, p. 64). Find out how long they have been with the department, which courses they teach, which committees they serve on, and what their research interests are. Ask each faculty member, "What do you wish you had known when you first became a faculty member?" or "What advice do you have for me?" Scheduling meetings with faculty likely will become more difficult as the semester progresses. Try to catch them in between semesters, or invite them to meet you sometime for coffee or lunch.

Staff

I learned through years of clinical work always to be kind and respectful to staff, regardless of their position or my position. When I worked at a hospital, I was proud that the housekeepers, house orderlies, and cafeteria workers knew my name. I would gladly stop and engage in a few minutes of friendly conversation with them. I continue to demonstrate that same level of respect in my academic role. I ask our administrative assistants how their kids and grandkids are doing or how they are coping with the medical treatments they are undergoing for a new diagnosis. I converse with our department's environmental services technician every day, enough to know that he is also an artist, just lost his father after a long battle with various health issues, and has worked at the university almost as long as I have been alive. Department staff often "hold more power than they are given credit for and can make things happen for you under the radar (e.g., expediting travel requests, ordering particular office supplies, securing an extra filing cabinet)" (Moe & Murphy, 2011, p. 65). Ask your department staff questions like, "Tell me about your responsibilities" and "What are some things that faculty do that annoy you?"

Administrators

Administrators like deans and provosts will not have time to meet with new faculty on an individual basis. You may have encountered them during the interview process, or you may go weeks or months without ever laying eyes on these upper-level administrators. However, you should be on the lookout for opportunities to meet them. As discussed earlier in this chapter, attend faculty meetings at the school and campus level whenever your schedule allows. Read your emails, and look for events where faculty are invited to interact with administrators. For example, I recently received an email inviting faculty to a "Coffee and Cookies with the Provost and

Chancellor" event. As a new faculty member, attending such an event may seem a little intimidating, but what do you have to lose? Go introduce yourself, explain that you are new to campus, and ask the administrators what they like best about the institution. Mingle with the few other individuals who showed up, add to your list of familiar faces on campus, and leave knowing that the administrator might just remember that someone from your specific department attended. Even better, find another new faculty member from your school to take with you so you have at least one other person with whom to chat comfortably.

ESTABLISHING YOUR REPUTATION

Krieger (2013) emphasized the importance of establishing your reputation during the first year. Watch what others are doing. Learn from your department chair and faculty colleagues. What are the formal expectations for when you should be in your office? Are there perhaps unspoken norms and flexibility about arrival and departure times? Which meetings and events are you expected to attend, and which ones will benefit you to attend even if they are not required? You may also consider spending a few extra hours in the office each week during your first few months to increase your visibility to students, faculty, and administrators (Moe & Murphy, 2011).

You also need to establish a reputation with your students. Students can sense the lack of experience of a new faculty member and will attack like sharks if they think you are not doing your job well enough. Start by laying out clear policies and course expectations and stick to them. One of the biggest mistakes you can make as a new faculty member is to make an exception for one student and not another, particularly when they are in a cohort-based program and know each other well. Word spreads quickly if you have been "unfair" by inconsistently enforcing course policies about attendance, late homework, etc. If you are teaching a cohort of students who have been in a professional program for a while and you are the new kid on the block, they may complain to other faculty about how your teaching approach is different than theirs. If word of this gets back to you, try not to take it personally. It is natural for students to resist change. It is natural for anyone to resist change. When I have encountered this situation, I addressed it briefly at the beginning of the next class period, explaining that each faculty member has a different style and encouraging students to come speak to me directly if they have concerns about my course. Likewise, you may encounter students who make negative comments to you about other faculty within your department. Again, remind students that it is much more professional of them to take up concerns about another course with that particular instructor.

Perhaps the two most important things you can do with students are convey to them that you have their learning as your highest priority and that you are there to support them. I always explain to students that just as they are on a journey to become an occupational therapist, I am on a journey to become a better occupational therapy educator. I explain that sometimes we will try new teaching and learning strategies, and sometimes they will not work out as planned. I explain not only what we are doing in a given class period but also why we are doing it. I try to learn their names, and I try to create a fun and friendly learning environment. I often arrive to class early and ask about their weekends, discuss the latest sports scores, or show a funny YouTube video before class just to set a positive tone before class. I frequently remind them of the course objectives, which in my profession are tied closely to standards set by an accrediting body for education programs. I give the cohort positive feedback throughout the course, particularly when I see a progression in critical thinking or their ability to apply what they are learning in concurrent coursework to an assignment in my course. I also let them know when I am disappointed in their performance or their professional behaviors, tying it directly back to how it reflects on them as future health care professionals. Of course, you want students to like you and your course, but chances are at least a few students will be upset about something and will make sure you hear about it in your end-of-course evaluations. Krieger (2013) reminded faculty that "the sign of teaching excellence is the performance of your students, and not only or mainly your students' satisfaction" (p. 146).

LEARNING ACTIVITIES

1. Explore the state-level governance structure of public institutions in your state on the website for the Education Commission of the States (www.ecs.org). Compare your findings to at least one other state.
2. Look for an organizational chart for a particular institution in which you are interested to gain an understanding of the institutional governance structure. If an organizational chart is not available, can you create one based on information on the institutional website?
3. Can you locate any examples of shared governance at your selected institution? Is there a faculty senate, curriculum committee, policy committee, or other faculty governance structure?
4. Interview a higher education administrator. Discuss the organizational models you learned about in this chapter. Which model most closely reflects this administrator's experience with institutional organization?
5. Explore the institutional website, and search for recent news stories about the institution. What information can you find that tells you about the campus climate and culture?
6. Interview a faculty member. How did this person learn information about the institution when starting out as a new faculty member? Ask about perceptions regarding climate and culture. What advice does this individual have for you as a new faculty member?

7. Locate and review the mission statement of at least three institutions. If you already work at a particular institution or have one in mind, find the mission statement for that institution and other institutions in the same region or state. Now look at the mission statement of an institution in a different state or perhaps of a different institutional type. What differences can you identify? How might the mission statement of the institution affect your particular health professions department? Can you locate mission statements for a specific department in your discipline? Do you see connections between the institutional mission statement and the departmental mission statement?

8. Look for your institution's strategic plan. Review the plan and identify areas in which your particular department can help meet institutional goals.

9. Find out if there is a faculty union at your institution or other institutions in your state. What is the role of the union? What are some of the recent initiatives of the union? Can you locate any recent news stories about the faculty union?

10. Explore the institution's website and look for campus events that would be helpful for a new faculty member to attend. Are there any campus-wide faculty meetings or meet and greet events with campus administrators?

11. Look for your institution's campus rules and regulations. Familiarize yourself with the broad categories of information, and carefully review at least a few of the specific policies.

12. Find any department- or school-level faculty handbooks or policy manuals that might provide additional guidance for faculty members. Which policies seem most relevant to you as a new faculty member?

13. Explore the website of a department in which you would like to work. What information can you gather about the faculty and staff in the department? Make a list of a few questions that you would ask if you had the opportunity to meet with each person briefly.

14. Familiarize yourself with campus resources available to faculty, staff, and students. These may include, but are not limited to, a counseling center, disability center, academic success center, career center, international center, center for teaching and learning, women's center, LGBTQ center, veterans center, library resources, and technology resources.

REFERENCES

American Association of University Professors. (n.d.a). *AAUP unionism.* Retrieved from https://www.aaupcbc.org/organize/aaup-unionism

American Association of University Professors. (n.d.b). *Shared governance.* Retrieved from https://www.aaup.org/our-programs/shared-governance

American Association of University Professors. (1966). *Statement on government of colleges and universities.* Retrieved from https://www.aaup.org/report/statement-government-colleges-and-universities

American Association of University Professors. (2010, March 25). *Faculty unions and governance: CBC Executive Committee comment on the AGB Statement on Institutional Governance.* Retrieved from https://www.aaup.org/news/faculty-unions-and-governance

Birnbaum, R. (1988). *How colleges work: The cyberkinetics of academic organization and leadership.* San Francisco, CA: Jossey-Bass.

Brock, D., & Symington, S. (2018). Effective ways to promote scholarship: The academic scholarship portfolio. In G. Kayingo & V. M. Hass (Eds.), *The health professions educator: A practical guide for new and established faculty* (pp. 263-274). New York, NY: Springer Publishing Company.

Buller, J. L. (2012). *The essential department chair: A comprehensive desk reference* (2nd ed.). San Francisco, CA: Jossey-Bass.

Carpenter-Hubin, J., & Snover, L. (2013). Key leadership positions and performance expectations. In P. J. Schloss & K. M. Cragg (Eds.), *Organization and administration in higher education* (pp. 27-49). New York, NY: Routledge.

Colton, J. (2007). The role of the department in the groves of academe. In A. L. Deneef & C. D. Goodwin (Eds.), *The academic's handbook* (3rd ed., pp. 367-386). Durham, NC: Duke University Press.

Education Commission of the States. (2018). *50-state comparison: State postsecondary governance structures.* Retrieved from https://www.ecs.org/50-state-comparison-postsecondary-governanc-structures

Hassanien, M. A. (2017). Strategic planning in higher education: A need for innovative model. *Journal of Education, Society, and Behavioural Science, 23*(2), 1-11. doi:10.9734/JESBS/2017/37428

HigherEdJobs. (2012). *What does the history of faculty unions teach us about their future?* Retrieved from https://www.higheredjobs.com/HigherEdCareers/interviews.cfm?ID=315

Kezar, A. (2012). Needed policies, practices, and values: Creating a culture to support and professionalize non-tenure track faculty. In A. Kezar (Ed.) *Embracing non-tenure track faculty: Changing campuses for the new faculty majority* (pp. 2-27). New York, NY: Routledge.

Krieger, M. H. (2013). *The scholar's survival manual.* Bloomington, IN: Indiana University Press.

Manning, K. (2013). *Organizational theory in higher education.* New York, NY: Routledge.

Martin, R. H. (2012, October 30). ABCs of accommodations. *The New York Times.* Retrieved from https://www.nytimes.com/2012/11/04/education/edlife/guide-to-accommodations-for-college-students-with-disabilities.html

Melear, K. B. (2013). The role of internal governance, committees, and advisory groups. In P. J. Schloss & K. M. Cragg (Eds.), *Organization and administration in higher education* (pp. 50-65). New York, NY: Routledge.

Moe, A. M., & Murphy, L. M. (2011). Being a new faculty. In E. Lenning, S. Brightman, & S. Caringella (Eds.), *A guide to surviving a career in academia: Navigating the rites of passage.* New York, NY: Routledge.

Moraine Valley Community College. (2018). *Mission statement.* Retrieved from https://www.morainevalley.edu/about/mission-and-history/mission-statement

National Council on Disability. (2015, May 19). *Briefing paper: Reauthorization of the Higher Education Act (HEA): The implications for increasing employment for people with disabilities.* Retrieved from https://www.ncd.gov/publications/2015/05192015

Peterson, M. W., & Spencer, M. G. (1990). Understanding academic culture and climate. *New Directions for Institutional Research, 1990*(68), 3-18.

Project Kaleidoscope. (2009). Balancing your career & personal life. Swarthmore. Retrieved from https://www.swarthmore.edu/sites/default/files/assets/documents/faculty-diversity-excellence/BalancingCareer.pdf

Pye, A. K. (2007). University governance and autonomy. In A. L. Deneef & C. D. Goodwin (Eds.) *The academic's handbook* (3rd ed., pp. 349-366). Durham, NC: Duke University Press.

University of Missouri. (2018). *Mission statement.* Retrieved from https://www.umsystem.edu/ums/about/mission

8

The Faculty Role
Teaching and Beyond

If you have worked in a clinical or other practice setting, think back to your first job. Whether your first job was in a hospital, school, outpatient, or other setting, you probably went into that job with one primary expectation—"I'm going to work with clients." As time went on, you likely learned that your position included a lot more than just direct client contact. There were staff meetings, documentation, quarterly or annual performance reviews, committees, leadership expectations, promotion opportunities, professional development opportunities, and countless other things that took up your time beyond working with your clients. Chances are that a lot of what you experienced during your first year surprised you.

Transitioning into an academic position can be much the same. You may enter the job thinking, "I'm going to teach students to become the next generation of practitioners in my profession," and you will, but there is so much more to the faculty role than just teaching. During my first year as a full-time faculty member, I was expected to teach two or three courses per semester. My initial naive thought was "What am I supposed to do with the rest of my time?!" I quickly realized how much time goes into course preparation, planning and carrying out learning activities, grading student work, advising students, attending meetings, and countless other activities that I did not know would be part of my academic job. This chapter explores the expectations of the faculty role beyond teaching. If you are preparing to pursue a faculty role, these are issues that you should bring up during the interview process to gain a better understanding of the specific expectations of the faculty position to which you are applying.

Railsback (1998), in response to a campus administrator who suggested that faculty only work about 200 hours per year (the time spent in the classroom), developed a list of the many other things that faculty do. "Just as it takes months to make a

Gateley, C. A. *Clinical Practice to Academia: A Guide for New and Aspiring Health Professions Faculty* (pp. 99-120). © 2021 Taylor & Francis Group.

two-hour movie or to prepare for a day-long courtroom appearance, the work behind the scenes at academic institutions goes far beyond what happens at the front of a classroom" (Railsback, 1998, para. 12). I will use the following list from Railsback's "The Duties of Professors at Colleges and Universities" as a general guide to organize the remainder of this chapter, with a few modifications based on my own experience as a non–tenure-track health professions faculty member:

- Work directly related to classroom teaching
- Other work related to teaching
- Service to students and colleagues
- Teaching and mentoring of graduate students
- Scholarship activities
- Service to your department, college, or university
- Service to one's field of study
- Service to the public

WORK DIRECTLY RELATED TO CLASSROOM TEACHING

Unless you are hired into a position with primary responsibilities of research or coordination of clinical sites, it is likely that your teaching responsibilities will demand your immediate attention (Moe & Murphy, 2011). If not provided to you, ask for copies of old syllabi and textbooks from previous instructors of the course or department staff who likely have access to such materials. Figure out which accreditation standards you are responsible for meeting in your particular course, and talk to your department chair and colleagues about how your course fits into the overall curriculum of the program. You will need to develop or revise a syllabus; select textbooks or other reading assignments; plan lectures, labs, and other in-class learning activities; and develop exams, assignments, and grading rubrics for those assignments.

Throughout the semester, you will need to plan and carry out activities for each class period, grade assignments, enter grades into the learning management system, respond to countless emails from students about absences and other issues, meet with students outside of class for help understanding material and assignments, and make adjustments to the course based on student learning. As you progress through the semester, keep notes about what worked well and what you should change the next time you teach the course. This is particularly helpful if the course is only taught one time per year and you will not be revising the course for several months. You may be asked to develop new courses, in which you are starting with a blank slate. Again, do not work in isolation. Seek guidance from your department colleagues and think about how the new course complements the existing curriculum.

OTHER WORK RELATED TO TEACHING

In addition to all the duties directly related to teaching described earlier, you may have other responsibilities indirectly related to teaching. For example, you may need to schedule and chaperone a field trip for your students to a local community agency that serves individuals with disabilities so students can learn their role in connecting their future clients with such resources. You may be responsible for coordinating and supervising teaching assistants for your courses. You may be asked to provide a peer review of teaching for a faculty colleague in your department or school. In turn, you may need to gather materials for other faculty to evaluate your own teaching. It is very likely that you will need to locate and arrange for guest lecturers to present information to your students in areas in which you are not an expert. These are just a few examples of the many responsibilities that go into planning and carrying out your teaching responsibilities.

SERVICE TO STUDENTS AND COLLEAGUES

Advising Students

When I first entered my faculty role, I did not have a complete understanding of what my role was in student advising. I vaguely remembered having to meet with someone before being allowed to register for courses during my first few years of college; however, once I entered my professional program, my cohort moved through a set curriculum, so there was no longer a need for discussing which courses I needed to take. I realize now that student advising involves so much more than simply recommending coursework. Your advising duties will differ greatly depending on the size and format of your program, but some common issues that you may face follow.

Advising Preprofessional Students

Your program may receive requests from high school students who are visiting campus and want to meet with someone from the department of their intended major. These appointments may be coordinated through your campus admissions department, and your advising appointment will likely be one item on the student's busy agenda that includes a campus tour and meetings with representatives from admissions, financial aid, and student affairs. Keep in mind that in most cases you will be meeting with the student and the family. Even though the parents may try to lead the discussion, I recommend that you speak directly to the student. You certainly need to answer questions that the family may have, but you should direct the conversation back to the student. This is a good time for students to learn that they have autonomy in determining their future academic paths and careers.

Your department may have a standard informational packet of materials including information about your profession, prerequisites, and guidelines for applying to the program. Here are some good questions to start out with that will help you determine which information to cover during the meeting:

- Tell me where you are in your college decision process. Are you exploring many campuses, or are you fairly certain this is where you plan to attend?
- Tell me where you are in the decision process about your major. Are you exploring other health professions, or are you fairly certain this discipline is what you want to pursue?
- Tell me what you already know about this discipline. Have you done any observations with someone in the field? Do you have a friend or family member that works in this profession or has received services from this profession?

As you ask these questions, assure the student and family that it is great to be exploring multiple campuses and majors as a high school junior or senior. Think back to when you were 17 years old. What did you envision for your future? Is that where you are now? What changed your educational and career path? High school students are under a lot of pressure from parents and society in general to have a clear plan about their futures (College Board, 2019). However, many students enter college undecided on a major or change their major at least once (Lieberman, 2017; National Center for Education Statistics, 2017). In high school, I always thought I would go into nursing. Then, in an act of rebellion against always doing what was expected of me, I entered college as a broadcast journalism major before eventually finding my way to occupational therapy. I hear similar stories from students all the time. Many students grew up knowing only about nursing or medicine or perhaps physical therapy and athletic training from an injury sustained during school sports. Have you ever heard a 10-year-old declare a desire to become a respiratory therapist, diagnostic medical ultrasonographer, or nuclear medicine technologist? Most students do not discover some of these lesser known health professions until they participate in a health professions career exploration course or have a family member who received services from these professions, so it is not unusual for students to be uncertain if your health profession is the right career path for them.

Part of your role in advising preprofessional students and their families is to help them gain a better understanding of the profession in general; what it takes to become a practitioner in your discipline; and what to expect in professional coursework, clinical placements (if applicable), and the entry-level job market. The following are some general topics that you should cover in a preprofessional advising appointment:

- A general overview of the profession
- What type of degree is required for entry-level practice?
- Is there a national board examination that must be passed?
- In what practice settings do professionals in your field work?
- Are there any specialty areas of practice? Do these specialty areas require advanced education?

- What is the job market outlook for your profession? What kind of salary can students expect? (Hint: You can find this information through your national professional association and the *Occupational Outlook Handbook* from the U.S. Department of Labor's Bureau of Labor Statistics at www.bls.gov/ooh)
- What is the educational pathway to obtaining a degree in your field? What prerequisite coursework is required? Is the admissions process competitive?

The answer to that last question often surprises many students and families. They may have come to their meeting with you thinking that they simply need to declare their major as physical therapy, pharmacy, or respiratory therapy and then take the required courses. Many health professions programs now have highly competitive admissions processes and receive three to four times the number of applications than available spots in the program. Students and families need to understand this reality. Give them the information that they need to make informed decisions and to maximize their chances of being accepted into a professional program. What factors play an important role in selecting applicants for your program? Is it grade point average (GPA)? The number of observation hours with professionals in your discipline? Leadership and involvement in community service? Advise them about campus resources that may be beneficial to them when they are applying to your program. The exact names of departments may vary by institution, but the following are a few general examples:

- Academic advising: Depending on the size and structure of your campus, academic advising of preprofessional students may fall to faculty in your department or to a separate office of professional advisors. In either case, encourage students to develop and maintain close connections to their advisors to stay abreast of academic requirements for particular health professions programs of interest to them.
- Campus career center: Most campuses have a department that helps students with exploring career options, building a résumé, writing personal statements for applications, and completing mock interviews.
- Student ambassadors: Many departments or health professions schools have students involved in professional coursework designated to serve as peer advisors to students interested in pursuing a career in a particular discipline. Encourage students to reach out to these ambassadors to help them answer questions that may arise about the application process. Depending on your institution's policies, you may be able to pass along the student's contact information directly to your school's student ambassadors so that they can reach out to the prospective student.
- Academic support center: Many college-bound students, particularly those with a history of academic success, are not used to asking for help. They may be unaware of campus resources available to them, such as writing labs, study groups, and free tutoring for challenging subjects. I emphasize to students and families that using these resources is not a sign of weakness but rather an excellent way to maximize academic performance. Most health professions programs have a minimum GPA requirement for admission, so students need information about how to succeed in their prerequisite coursework.

- Office of student services: These departments can help connect students to organizations that give them opportunities for campus involvement and leadership. You may also have information about student organizations specific to your discipline or health professions in general that you can pass on to students. I remind students that it looks better on an application to be an involved member of one or two organizations rather than an uninvolved member of five or more organizations.

- Office of community engagement: Many students enter college with a history of volunteerism. The importance of community engagement has been instilled in them from a young age. Most college and scholarship applications ask students to list service activities in which they have been involved (Barge, 2018). There is a good chance that this is also a factor in the application process to your specific program. Students and families often want to know which volunteer opportunities exist on your campus or in your community for students, particularly if they are moving to an unfamiliar area. In addition to the campus resources available, be sure to share with students any information you have about opportunities that may look particularly good on an application to your program.

- Office of disability services: More students are entering college with a history of physical, emotional, or learning disabilities that may impact their academic performance (Kutscher, Naples, & Freund, 2019). Although students and families may be hesitant to disclose this information in an initial advising meeting, you can simply include information about this office in your overview of available campus services.

In addition to high school students, you may also be responsible for the advisement of preprofessional students already enrolled on your campus. They may be interested in changing majors or clarifying details about an upcoming application process. For these students, simply start out with general questions such as "Tell me about yourself" and "What can I answer for you today?" to get a sense of which topics you should cover during your appointment.

Advising Professional Students

In many health professions programs, students are assigned a faculty advisor from their respective programs once they enter the professional phase of their coursework. Unless your department has some established guidelines for advising, you may be a little uncertain regarding your advising role with these students. When I started my first full-time faculty position, I inherited some advisees who previously had been assigned to a recent retiree. Within the first few months in my new faculty position, I had to meet with multiple advisees about issues such as academic performance below department standards, academic dishonesty (in this case plagiarism), and professional behavior concerns including excessive absences and tardiness to class. Those meetings were not pleasant experiences for me or the students. I realized that I never again wanted my first advising appointment with a student to be centered on a negative issue.

Although it was not required, I made a point to schedule a brief advising appointment with each of my advisees every semester in order for us to get to know each other better. Because their coursework was already predetermined, I focused first-time meetings on learning more about them and helping students understand the expectations of our program in terms of academic performance and professional behavior. I also made sure they had a clear understanding of upcoming coursework and fieldwork. Students may be intimidated by you initially, so start out by asking open-ended questions such as "How are things going this semester?" and "What else are you involved in outside of class?" Many students are balancing several extracurricular activities, employment, family responsibilities, and other life roles. Students are often surprised at the academic rigor of professional programs in comparison to their general education and prerequisite courses. You may need to help them recognize the need to prioritize their commitments and give up one or more outside commitments to ensure their academic success in your program.

As students advance through your program, your advising sessions should become more like comfortable conversations. Students may ask advice about a challenging situation they are having with a particular classmate or professor. Be careful that you do not get lured into saying something negative about a colleague. Instead, encourage the student to approach that particular faculty member with his or her concerns. Students may ask for your recommendation about options for upcoming clinical placements, studying for a board exam, or employment searches. They may also open up to you about issues they are dealing with in their personal lives, such as anxiety, depression, grief, and relationship issues. Although you should provide general emotional support, do not take it upon yourself to act as the student's personal counselor. Make sure you are well informed about campus resources and be ready to provide information to students and encourage them to seek out the help they need.

Letters of Recommendation

Have you ever asked someone for a letter of recommendation when you were applying for a scholarship, professional program, job, or other opportunity? You were probably appreciative of their time and effort, but other than a simple "thank you" there was no way to repay the favor. As a faculty member, you will have the opportunity to pay it forward many times over. Students and colleagues may call on you to write letters of support for opportunities they are pursuing.

Students

I get asked to write approximately 10 letters of recommendation per semester for students applying for scholarships and leadership opportunities. Students typically contact me by email or ask me in person before or after class. Although I have no limit to the total number of letters I will write in a given semester, I have established a rule that I will only write two letters for the same scholarship or opportunity. I believe that anything beyond that starts to look disingenuous to the committee reviewing applications and letters. I communicate this guideline to my advisees and students in my courses so they know to ask me sooner rather than later for a recommendation letter. When I agree to write a letter, I ask the student to email me a current résumé and information about the scholarship or opportunity so I can individualize the recommendation letter. When feasible for our schedules, I also find it helpful to discuss with the students in person or via phone their reasons for applying and why they think they are good candidates.

I keep an electronic file of all the recommendation letters I have written over the years. It helps to have a general template with which to start, and then I add in details specific to the student and criteria for the scholarship or leadership opportunity. If the criteria for the scholarship include academic achievement, leadership involvement, and service to others, be sure to include information in the letter about each factor. If a leadership opportunity requires exceptional interpersonal and organization skills, give specific examples of the student's performance in these areas. Also, be sure you know how the letter should be delivered. Does it need to be returned directly to the student? Does it need to be sent directly to a selection committee? Does it need to be in written or electronic format? If written format is required, does it need to be on department letterhead and in a sealed envelope with your signature over the seal? Regardless of the delivery method, I always provide the student with an electronic copy of what I have written. If you are not comfortable with the student reading what you wrote, you probably should not have agreed to write the recommendation in the first place. See Box 8-1 for a sample letter of recommendation for a student.

Colleagues

In addition to recommendation letters for students, I occasionally get asked to provide letters of recommendation or support for colleagues pursuing promotion or professional leadership and development opportunities. Much like the student letters of recommendation, I find it helpful to have a copy of the individual's current curriculum vitae and specific information about the criteria for the opportunity he or she is pursuing. See Box 8-2 for an example of a recommendation letter for a professional colleague.

Employment References for Students

As students approach the end of their coursework and clinical rotations in your program, they are likely to ask their professors and advisors to serve as employment references as they pursue entry-level employment. Although a few smaller employers still make direct phone calls to check references, many larger companies have transitioned to using a brief online survey to gather information about applicants. In addition to several Likert ratings, these surveys have an option to add in a narrative response about the applicant's strengths and areas for improvement. Most of the online reference checks that I have completed for students and recent graduates took only about 5 minutes to complete.

Dear School of Health Professions Ambassador Selection Committee:

I am writing this letter to recommend Ms. Jenna Burns for the SHP Ambassador and Leadership Program. I am an instructor in the Department of Occupational Therapy, and I have had the pleasure of having Jenna in class during the Fall 2019 semester.

Jenna is an excellent student. She finished her undergraduate coursework with a 4.0 cumulative GPA, and she currently has a 3.85 cumulative GPA in our professional program. Jenna has been the recipient of several academic scholarships and honors including the University of Missouri Excellence Award, Bright Flight Scholarship, SHarP Scholars Scholarship, and the Dean's List. She is also a pleasure to have in class, often contributing to class discussion and asking insightful questions.

Beyond her strong academic credentials, Jenna also has demonstrated a commitment to serving others through a number of employment and volunteer activities. She has worked as a therapy technician at a local rehabilitation hospital and is therefore familiar with a number of health professions beyond her chosen career in occupational therapy. Jenna has also gained valuable experience working with individuals with different abilities through her position as a proctor with the Office of Disability Services. In addition, Jenna has been very active in campus and community organizations throughout her high school and college years and has held a number of leadership positions.

In summary, I believe Jenna's combination of scholastic achievement, work experience in service-oriented positions, and leadership in campus and community activities makes her an excellent candidate for the SHP Ambassador and Leadership Program. I believe she would do a fantastic job of representing the SHP at recruitment, alumni, and public relations events. I strongly recommend her for this opportunity.

Sincerely,

Crystal A. Gateley, PhD, OTR/L

555-555-5555

crystalgateley@myuniversity.edu

Box 8-1. Sample letter of recommendation for student.

Before completing letters of recommendation or employment references for students, check with department administrators to ensure that you are abiding by the Family Educational Rights and Privacy Act and following any departmental or institutional restrictions regarding the release of information. You may need to have students sign a release of information form or keep record of their requests for you to complete letters of recommendation or employment references.

To Whom It May Concern:

This letter is intended to serve as a recommendation for Jamie Stephens as a candidate for the Doctor of Philosophy in Pediatric Science degree program at Rocky Mountain University. I have had the privilege of knowing Jamie for nearly 12 years. I first met her in 2007 at Lewis & Clark Rehabilitation Center in Columbia, MO. She was a staff physical therapist in the outpatient department where I served as Director of Outpatient Therapy. We later worked together as colleagues at Mid-Missouri Hospital in Columbia, MO. Although we have since moved on to different positions, we have maintained frequent contact at both a professional and personal level. I therefore believe that I can provide you with the information you are seeking about Jamie as a potential candidate for your program.

I imagine that all of your applicants have exceptional backgrounds in clinical skills and work experience, and Jamie is no exception. However, I believe what makes Jamie an excellent candidate for your graduate program is her love for learning and her ongoing commitment to professional advancement. Throughout her professional career, Jamie has consistently sought out professional development opportunities, often at considerable cost and personal time. Beyond the standard weekend continuing education courses in which most physical therapists engage, she also completed lengthy certification trainings in Neuro-Developmental Treatment in 2002 and 2003. More recently, Jamie completed a distance education post-professional Doctorate of Physical Therapy (DPT) degree, and she did so while successfully balancing full-time work and family responsibilities. Furthermore, she completed her DPT program with the same academic excellence she has demonstrated throughout her academic career.

Jamie has aspirations of teaching at a research university, and she recognizes that obtaining her PhD in Pediatric Science is the next step to achieving that goal. I am in the midst of pursuing a PhD myself, and Jamie and I have had numerous conversations about the joys and frustrations of graduate coursework. She recognizes the challenges that lie ahead if she is accepted into your program, and I have no doubt that she will be successful in this endeavor. She is blessed with a supportive family who provide her with the encouragement and logistical help necessary to balance work, school, and family responsibilities.

In summary, Jamie has as much to offer academia as she does to gain from it. I believe you will find her to be an excellent student, and she wants to become an excellent researcher as well. It is without reservation that I recommend Jamie Stephens as a candidate for the Doctor of Philosophy in Pediatric Science degree program.

Respectfully,

Crystal A. Gateley, PhD, OTR/L

555-555-5555

crystalgateley@myuniversity.edu

Box 8-2. Sample recommendation for professional colleague.

TEACHING AND MENTORING OF GRADUATE STUDENTS

If your professional program is at the graduate level, you may be responsible for teaching and mentoring students through advanced coursework, research, clinicals, and other experiential learning. Some health professions programs have teaching clinics as part of their academic program, through which community members receive clinical services while students get the opportunity to develop their skills under the close supervision of faculty. Many graduate-level health professions programs encourage or require their students to engage in research activities, so you may be responsible for mentoring students through the entire research process from proposal development to institutional review board (IRB) approval to presentation of research findings via professional conferences and publications. Depending on the requirements of your program, you may also be responsible for evaluating the proposals and defenses of graduate student theses, dissertations, or capstone projects.

SCHOLARSHIP ACTIVITIES

Railsback (1998) originally referred to this category as "research activities." I have used the broader term of *scholarship activities* because even if traditional research is not an expectation of your faculty position, you may still be expected to engage in other forms of scholarship. At minimum, you may be expected to keep abreast of recent developments in your discipline by reading scholarly journals and attending conferences of your state and national professional association. As you gain more experience in your faculty role, you may be expected to submit proposals for posters and presentations at such conferences. A few things to consider related to scholarship expectations follow.

Research

If research is part of your workload distribution, you will need to explore resources far beyond this textbook for guidance with obtaining funding and IRB approval for research. Your institution likely will have an IRB office and some type of support for grant writing. Crossland (2007) listed several common sources of grant funding, including your own institution, public sources, private individuals and corporations, nonprofit agencies, government agencies, and broad-based philanthropies and foundations. Watch your emails closely for announcements about upcoming funding opportunities. In addition to a budget of how you will spend awarded grant money, grant applications should include a thorough description of the problem and gaps in knowledge about the problem, an explanation of how your research will provide a unique contribution to better understand or address the problem, and a persuasive argument about the overall potential impact of your research (Krieger, 2013). Your institution may have individuals who are experienced in grant writing who can help guide your grant proposal to ensure appropriate content and structure. Larger institutions typically have one or more people whose specific job it is to assist with grants. If this is the case at your institution, watch for advertisements about upcoming informational sessions and other trainings provided by this office. Krieger (2013) explained that minor mistakes, such as spelling and grammatical errors, inconsistent formatting, or the use of incorrect technical terms, are "credibility killers" in grant proposals (p. 175). If you want to pursue research and do not know much about the process, I recommend you find yourself an experienced mentor who can guide you through your first few research endeavors.

Scholarship Beyond Basic Research

Boyer (1990) proposed the following broadened definition of scholarship that recognizes the reciprocal relationship between theory and practice:

> Theory surely leads to practice. But practice also leads to theory. And teaching, at its best, shapes both research and practice. Viewed from this perspective, a more comprehensive, more dynamic understanding of scholarship can be considered, one in which the rigid categories of teaching, research, and service are broadened and more flexibly defined. (p. 16)

Boyer (1990) proposed the following model of scholarship:

- Scholarship of discovery: Basic research that advances knowledge
- Scholarship of integration: Synthesis of knowledge from different disciplines
- Scholarship of application: Use of knowledge to address societal problems
- Scholarship of teaching: Exploration of theory and practice related to teaching and learning, also known as scholarship of teaching and learning

Health professions faculty have the opportunity to engage in all forms of scholarship described by Boyer. New faculty should seek out mentorship from more experienced colleagues to develop projects, collect data, and report findings through publication or presentation.

Publishing

If you are conducting any kind of scholarship, you should consider publishing your work. Most health professions have at least one peer-reviewed journal and one practice magazine specific to the discipline. "In academic publishing, the goal of peer review is to assess the quality of articles submitted for publication in a scholarly journal" (City University of New York, 2018, para. 1). Authors submit an article to a journal editor who then forwards the article to other experts in the field to evaluate the quality of the manuscript.

> The peer reviewers check the manuscript for accuracy and assess the validity of the research methodology and procedures. If appropriate, they suggest revisions. If they find the article lacking in scholarly validity and rigor, they reject it. Because a peer-reviewed journal will not publish articles that fail to meet the standards established for a given discipline, peer-reviewed articles that are accepted for publication exemplify the best research practices in a field. (City University of New York, 2018, para. 2)

Examples of peer-reviewed journals in the health professions include *Respiratory Care, Journal of Diagnostic Medical Sonography, Journal of Athletic Training,* and *American Journal of Audiology.* In contrast to peer-reviewed journals, practice magazines typically contain articles of clinical interest, news about the profession, advertisements for products, continuing education opportunities, and job openings. Examples of discipline-specific practice magazines include *Orthopaedic Physical Therapy Practice, OT Practice,* and *The ASHA Leader.* Although any published work helps build your curriculum vitae, publishing in peer-reviewed journals will be more valued when your dossier is being reviewed for promotion or tenure. You should seek guidance from your department chair, colleagues, and other mentors about which publications are most appropriate for your work (Moe & Murphy, 2011).

If you have a particular area of expertise within your discipline, you may be able to publish a chapter in a textbook, or perhaps even an entire textbook, about that topic. Getting into this type of publishing often starts with a connection to someone who is already involved in publishing. Never would I have imagined that I would be authoring textbooks about occupational therapy or the health professions. However, a former professor of mine had published a textbook on clinical documentation. She retired from her academic position after the second edition of the textbook was published, and she asked if I would be interested in coauthoring the third edition of the textbook with her. I was reluctant at first because I knew absolutely nothing about the publishing process, but she and the editors were very supportive and guided me through the process.

Although having a connection in the industry is helpful, there are other ways to get started with textbook publishing. If you have an idea for a chapter or a book, contact a publishing company in your discipline to discuss your idea with an acquisitions editor. That individual can give you a sense if your idea is something in which the company would even be interested. You will need to write up a proposal for the project that includes, at minimum, a description of the project, the target audience and potential buyers, competitors (if any), a table of contents, and a projected timeline of completion. If you are unknown to the publishing company, they may want a sample of your work, such as a few chapters from the proposed book or other project. Some publishers may have very specific formats for book proposals that you will need to follow. Be sure to explore the website for submission guidelines (Davidson & Wissoker, 2007). Beyond emails and phone calls, talking with representatives from textbook publishing companies at your national professional conferences is another great way to get your foot in the door of the publishing industry. Again, it is always helpful to have a mentor who can guide you through the process.

If you are submitting a proposal for an article, chapter, book, or other publishing project, you need to be prepared for rejection or considerable revision. You will be getting feedback from peer reviewers and editors, and you will need to respond to each piece of feedback by making revisions or by justifying why you chose not to make a revision. "Sometimes these reviews are wonderfully helpful, sometimes they are neutral, and more often than is desirable, they may be insulting and hurtful or misunderstanding or nitpicky or pushing you in peculiar directions" (Krieger, 2013, p. 75). Publishing is a great learning experience, and it certainly will give you more empathy for students who are upset or frustrated by feedback from you when you grade their assignments.

Presenting

In addition to publishing, conducting presentations at local, state, national, and international conferences is another great way to share your scholarly work with others. Conferences typically send out a call for proposals several months in advance of the event, with guidelines for submission of proposed workshops, sessions, and posters. If you are unfamiliar with these types of presentations, be sure to attend a professional conference for your discipline, and explore the different types of presentations that you may be interested in doing in the future. If your submission is selected for presentation at the conference, you will need to spend time preparing for the presentation. If you are presenting a poster, the conference coordinators will have specific guidelines for you regarding the size of the poster and how it will be displayed. If you are presenting a workshop or other type of session, you will need to follow guidelines regarding time allotment and audiovisual equipment. Many conferences now encourage presenters to upload their handouts well in advance of the conference so that interested attendees may access them electronically before and during the event.

SERVICE TO YOUR DEPARTMENT, COLLEGE, OR UNIVERSITY

There are numerous ways in which you will spend time serving your department, your division, and your campus (Railsback, 1998). You will spend countless hours each year attending department-, school-, and campus-level meetings. You also may be expected to attend convocation and commencement exercises. Over the years, I have heard many faculty members grumble about having to give up a weekend day to attend graduation. Attending graduation is one of my favorite parts of my job. This is why we do what we do! Of course, I want to see the students I have taught over the past few years achieve such an important milestone in their lives. There are 104 Saturdays and Sundays each year. I do not mind spending 2 of those days, once for spring graduation and once for fall graduation, celebrating my students' accomplishments. Particularly in small cohort programs where students and faculty know each other well, students may be disappointed when one or more professors are absent on their important day.

Service on Formal Committees

Faculty members are often assigned to one or more committees at the department and school levels. As you gain more experience, you may also be asked to serve on a campus-level committee. Most committees have rotating membership. For example, a school-level curriculum committee may have 6 members, each serving staggered 3-year terms. When new members join the committee, there are always members on the committee who have more experience and can guide new members about the committee's expectations and responsibilities. Committees often elect a new chair each academic year. Unless someone is eager to serve in this leadership role, this topic typically leads to a group of faculty sitting around a conference room table either refusing to make eye contact with each other or immediately providing reasons why they cannot take on the responsibility. If you are in academia for more than a few years, it is almost inevitable that you will need to take a turn serving in a committee leadership role.

You may also be asked to serve on search committees for faculty and staff positions. As a newer faculty member, you likely will be asked to serve on such committees only at the department level. Within a few years, you may be asked to serve on search committees at the school and campus levels as well. Search committees typically involve a short-term commitment because once someone is hired for the position, the committee disbands. However, some searches, particularly at the school and campus levels, can last several months until the right person for the position is identified and hired.

Participation in School and Campus Events

Beyond convocation and commencement exercises, you may be asked to represent your department at various school and campus events. For example, each summer my school of health professions hosts a 2-day event to introduce high school students from underprivileged backgrounds to health professions careers, and faculty are asked to volunteer to represent their disciplines and facilitate hands-on learning activities for the students. Faculty also get asked to serve on faculty panels during summer orientation and welcome week activities to discuss the transition to college with students and parents. Another example of service that you may be asked to perform is representing your department at school- or campus-level fairs introducing students to particular majors and careers.

Faculty Mentor to Student Groups

At most institutions, student groups require a faculty mentor in order to be officially recognized as a campus organization. Most health professions programs have some sort of student organization, either specific to the discipline or perhaps general to the health professions. As a faculty mentor, you will be expected to attend meetings and guide the student leaders in planning activities and events.

Selecting Students for Your Professional Program

If you take a faculty position, it is very likely that you will be involved in the process of selecting students for your professional program. This may involve reviewing applications, résumés, and personal essays or conducting individual or group interviews with applicants. Most health professions programs now have a very competitive application process and receive upwards of three to four times the number of applications in comparison to the number of slots they have available in the program. If you are applying for a faculty position, find out information about the program's application and admissions process. Explore the program's website first. Depending on what information you can find online, consider asking your potential employer the following questions:

- How many students do you accept each year?
- How many applications do you receive each year?
- What are your criteria for applicants?
- Do you have a set application deadline or do you accept applications on a rolling basis?
- How are faculty involved in the selection process?
- What attracts students to your professional program?

Coordinating Clinical Sites

Another responsibility you may encounter as a health professions faculty member is the need to recruit and maintain sufficient clinical sites for your students (Chastain, 2018). In some health professions programs, a faculty member may have responsibility for this task in addition to teaching and research expectations. Other programs may have a clinical or fieldwork coordinator whose primary role is establishing and maintaining relationships with clinical sites, which is not nearly as simple as it sounds. Both parties must come to an agreement, typically in the form of a legal contract, for the educational affiliation. In addition, the clinical coordinator for the academic program must coordinate student background screenings, immunizations, drug screenings, and numerous other details before a student can arrive at a clinical site. Depending on your profession, clinical sites may require that the academic program provide a preceptor when students are on site, while other professions expect that the clinical site will provide the preceptor, clinical instructor, fieldwork educator, or whatever the terminology is in your profession. Your profession likely has accreditation standards that further regulate clinical experiences in terms of length, setting, qualifications of sites and supervisors, and assessment of student performance. Additionally, there may be discipline-specific training that is either required or encouraged for clinicians to serve as clinical supervisors.

During my years in clinical practice, I often served as the fieldwork coordinator for students at the hospitals and outpatient clinics where I worked. Academic programs would contact me months, and sometimes years, in advance asking for a commitment from my department to take a student. At any given time, I was juggling requests from five to seven different educational programs across our region, and I had to plan carefully how many students we would be taking at any given time. When I was asked to make a commitment one or two years in advance, I honestly did not know who would even be working in my department at that time, much less if they would be qualified and willing to take a student. Perhaps the person I had planned to supervise the student would take another job elsewhere or be out on maternity leave. As a result, it is not uncommon for the clinical coordinators in academic programs to deal with last-minute cancellations of students' clinical rotations, which can be anxiety-provoking for both the clinical coordinator and the students affected. For over 10 years, I have watched the ongoing struggles of the clinical coordinators in my own program and across our School of Health Professions as they try to ensure adequate clinical placements for all their students and scramble to make adjustments when unexpected situations arise. "The key to success as a clinical coordinator is to have in place alternatives that allow students' clinical experiences to continue without delaying their matriculation" (Chastain, 2018, p. 122).

Beyond cancellations from the clinical sites, academic clinical coordinators also must manage the expectations and changing situations of their students. Students typically do not understand the monumental work of the clinical coordinator in establishing the list of clinical sites available to them. As the demand for health care providers continues to rise, the number and enrollment of health professions programs across the country have also increased, making it even more difficult for clinical coordinators to establish and maintain enough sites to serve all their students and allow for backup plans. In our academic program, we have fieldwork sites across our state, in neighboring states, and across the country. For shorter 1-week placements, the clinical coordinator takes student preference into account to some extent, but, ultimately, he assigns students to their locations. For longer placements, which in my program consist of two 12-week rotations, students complete a "preference sheet" indicating their top five choices for each rotation along with a statement about what is the single most important factor for them. For example, perhaps a student wants a pediatric rotation no matter what, and location is less of a concern. Another student, married with small children and a mortgage payment, may consider staying in the nearby area of utmost importance and be far less concerned with the clinical setting or patient population. The clinical coordinator then randomizes the student names and goes through the list trying to ensure that each student gets two placements that fall somewhere on his or her list of preferences.

Inevitably, one or more students will be upset about their assigned placements. I have seen students in tears or talking angrily with their peers or on their phones with their parents. I have seen GroupMe (Microsoft) texts where students complain incessantly about how "unfair" the process is. I have witnessed the end of close friendships because one student got the placement that the other student desperately wanted. Although our clinical coordinator, only somewhat jokingly, explains repeatedly to students that he is not their travel agent and that the ultimate goal is that they have a quality learning experience that prepares them for entry-level practice, some students always complain.

Every health professions program has a different method for determining student clinical placements. If this is not part of your job as a new faculty member, take time to talk with your program's clinical coordinator to learn more about how the process is handled in your particular program and how courses you teach are related to clinical experiences. How many contracts does your program have with clinical sites? How does the coordinator handle the process of assigning clinical placements? How is student performance assessed? How do accreditation standards influence the process? How will the courses you are responsible for teaching help prepare students for those clinical experiences?

SERVICE TO YOUR FIELD OF STUDY

In addition to service to your department, school, and campus, you may also be involved in service to your profession. Perhaps you serve on the state licensure board for your profession or have a leadership role in your state association. As you begin attending academic conferences and making connections in your profession at the national level, you may be asked to serve on national committees and task forces as well. Other examples of service to your field of study include reviewing submissions to academic journals and professional conferences, serving on editorial boards, and reviewing grant proposals submitted to funding agencies.

SERVICE TO THE PUBLIC

Your university, school, or program may have a commitment to community engagement in addition to its teaching and research missions. For example, a physical therapy department may host an annual fall prevention workshop and screening at a local senior center. An occupational therapy department may host a car seat fitting clinic or Backpack Awareness Day. A respiratory therapy department may provide a weekend camp for children to learn about how to manage their asthma. A school of health professions may hold community service days to benefit local organizations. In all of these examples, faculty participation is needed for successful planning and implementation. If you are applying for an academic position, search the department or school website for recent news stories about community engagement. Be sure to inquire about these opportunities and expectations during an interview.

CONCLUSION

This chapter highlighted some of the many expectations of faculty beyond the time spent directly in the classroom, particularly in regard to service activities. Some faculty may view service as simply one more responsibility added to an already busy schedule. I choose to view it as an opportunity to learn more about how academia works and to network with colleagues both internal and external to my profession. Additionally, service activities may be an expectation of your faculty role, and involvement and leadership in committee work look good on your curriculum vitae when you are seeking promotion. The following are some questions to ask during an interview about service expectations:

- What are the service expectations for this position?
- Which committees might I serve on in my first few years in this position?
- What opportunities are there for campus-level service?
- Tell me about the involvement of faculty in professional organizations at the state and national level.

Moe and Murphy (2011) recommended volunteering for service that you want to do before you get assigned to something you do not want to do. Additionally, they warned against the possibility of unfair expectations of service for minority faculty members.

> Beware of the potential ... for exploitation based on how your colleagues perceive you. If you are a minority in any way, be it by gender, race, ethnicity, sexual orientation, etc., you may find you are expected to assume more service or particular types of service. While such work might be the most meaningful to you ... it is ultimately unfair and discriminatory for you to be expected to do more because of your status or demographic. (Moe & Murphy, 2011, p. 71)

I want to conclude this chapter with a quote that resonated with me as I was exploring resources for this book. Sometimes we get so caught up in our many responsibilities as faculty members that we lose sight of why we chose college teaching as a career path. Hauerwas (2007) described how faculty members often forget that they are part of a larger institution and implored faculty to remember that the vocation of teaching is what gives them common ground.

> Most of us seldom feel like members of a university faculty. Instead we are members of department—those people who come the closest to understanding what we are about. After all, what do we have in common with someone from sociology, biochemistry, or theology? This feeling may well lead us to believe we have no responsibility to serve, for example, on university committees, except as such service is necessary either for tenure or the goodwill of our chairperson (which may be the same thing). Any sense that we are members of a community dedicated to the exploring and passing on of the wisdom of our culture seems to have been lost. What I am suggesting is that such a sense of community will not be regained unless we are able to recover the obvious, but no less important, realization that our first vocation as university people is to teach. That is what we share in common and what makes us part of a cooperative endeavor. (p. 41)

LEARNING ACTIVITIES

1. Locate a job announcement for a faculty position in your discipline. What duties are included in the description? What other activities from this chapter do you think the position might entail?

2. Interview a faculty member in the health professions. Ask about how the individual spends time outside of the classroom? What other activities is he or she responsible for. Compare responses with other classmates.

3. Think about a course you have taken at some point in your college career, preferably one for which you can still access the syllabus. What planning do you think went into developing the course? Now think about a course you may teach or assist with at some point in the future. What are some of the behind-the-scenes preparations you would need to complete in order for students to have a successful learning experience?

4. Reflect on academic advisors you have had throughout your college career. What role did they play in your academic journey? What are some positive and negative experiences that you had with them? What attributes would you like to exhibit as an advisor to students?

5. Explore the student support services available on your campus or at an institution where you hope to obtain a faculty position. What resources are available to students? Is there a fee for any of the services, or are these services already accounted for in general tuition and student fees? How easy was it to locate them on the institution's website? Which resources would be most important to educate current and future students about?

6. Explore the IRB requirements for your campus or one at which you hope to work. What type of training is required? Is training provided on an ongoing basis or only at certain times of the year? What is the process for obtaining IRB approval?

7. Explore the curricula vitae of faculty in a particular department. Look at their publications, presentations, and other scholarly activities. What forms of scholarship are they involved in?

8. What opportunities exist in your discipline for scholarship of teaching and learning? Does your profession have any specific initiatives or scholarship agendas related to teaching? Is there a particular academic journal or conference that focuses specifically on teaching in your discipline?

9. Explore the opportunities for publishing in your discipline. What are the primary academic journals for your profession? Are there practice magazines? Which companies publish textbooks for your profession? Can you locate any information about submission guidelines for any of these publication venues?

10. Explore the professional association meetings relevant for your profession, including local, state, regional, national, and international events. Recognizing that you may not be able to attend every event because of financial limitations, which events are most important to attend?

11. Find out which student groups are available on your campus for your particular discipline or for health professions students in general. Can you locate information about the faculty advisors for any of these groups? Consider reaching out to one or more of these individuals, and ask about the time commitment they have in mentoring the student group.

12. Explore the admissions practices for a particular program in your discipline. What factors are taken into consideration during the admissions process? Can you locate any information about acceptance rates?

13. Find out information about the clinical sites used by a particular academic program in your discipline. This information may not be readily available on department websites, so you may need to email or call someone involved in coordinating clinical sites to learn more about how clinical sites are determined.

14. Explore the leadership opportunities available in your discipline at the local, state, and national levels. Which elected or appointed positions exist? Are there any committees of particular interest to you?

15. Find out if your campus engages in any public service events relevant to health professions students and faculty.

REFERENCES

Barge, M. A. (2018, May 1). How many volunteer hours do you need for college? PrepScholar. Retrieved from https://blog.prepscholar.com/how-many-volunteer-hours-for-college

Boyer, E. L. (1990). *Scholarship reconsidered: Priorities of the professoriate.* Carnegie Foundation for the Advancement of Teaching. Retrieved from https://depts.washington.edu/gs630/Spring/Boyer.pdf

Chastain, A. P. (2018). Recruiting and maintaining clinical sites. In G. Kayingo & V. M. Hass (Eds.), *The health professions educator: A practical guide for new and established faculty* (pp. 121-130). New York, NY: Springer Publishing Company.

City University of New York. (2018). *Evaluating information sources: What is a peer-reviewed article?* Retrieved from https://guides.lib.jjay.cuny.edu/c.php?g=288333&p=1922599

College Board. (2019). *5 ways to find career ideas.* Retrieved from https://bigfuture.collegeboard.org/get-started/know-yourself/5-ways-to-find-career-ideas

Crossland, F. E. (2007). New academics and the quest for private funds. In A. L. Deneef & C. D. Goodwin (Eds.), *The academic's handbook* (3rd ed., pp. 278-290). Durham, NC: Duke University Press.

Davidson, C. N., & Wissoker, K. (2007). Academic book publishing. In A. L. Deneef & C. D. Goodwin (Eds.), *The academic's handbook* (3rd ed., pp. 315-333). Durham, NC: Duke University Press.

Hauerwas, S. M. (2007). The morality of teaching. In A. L. Deneef & C. D. Goodwin (Eds.), *The academic's handbook* (3rd ed., pp. 38-46). Durham, NC: Duke University Press.

Krieger, M. H. (2013). *The scholar's survival manual.* Bloomington, IN: Indiana University Press.

Kutscher, E., Naples, L., & Freund, M. (2019, March). *Students with disabilities and post-college employment: How much do we know?* National Center for College Students with Disabilities. Retrieved from http://www.nccsdonline.org/research-briefs.html

Lieberman, L. (2017, August 24). *Still undecided? Here's how to pick your college major.* Study Breaks. Retrieved from https://studybreaks.com/college/undecided-how-to-pick-college-major/

Moe, A. M., & Murphy, L. M. (2011). Being a new faculty. In E. Lenning, S. Brightman, & S. Caringella (Eds.), *A guide to surviving a career in academia: Navigating the rites of passage*. New York, NY: Routledge.

National Center for Education Statistics. (2017). *Beginning college students who change their majors within 3 years of enrollment*. Retrieved from https://nces.ed.gov/pubs2018/2018434.pdf

Railsback, B. (1998). The duties of professors at colleges and universities. Retrieved from http://www. gly.uga.edu/railsback/railsback_profduties.html

9

Understanding Today's College Students

Whether you are preparing for a full-time academic position, an adjunct instructor position, or even a role as an occasional guest lecturer, one of the first things you need to understand is that college students likely are not the same as they were when you attended college, whether that was just a few years ago or several decades ago. We know that, in general, most students attend college because they and their families understand that a college education will give them improved chances for a good career and a better life. Individuals with at least some level of postsecondary education significantly increase their lifetime earning potential, are healthier, and are more engaged in civic life (Merisotis, 2017). Yet, across higher education, only 25% of students are in a major with a well-defined career path (McGraw Hill Education, 2017). Most students pursuing a career in the health professions fall within that 25%. They know they want to be an ultrasonographer, athletic trainer, or respiratory therapist, and there is a clearly defined degree program and national board examination that they must complete to achieve their goal.

It seems simple, right? We, as educators, lay out a curriculum that meets accreditation standards and guide students through learning what they need to know for entry-level practice in their chosen profession. However, this approach assumes that all students enter our programs with the same level of knowledge, skills, and desire to meet our expectations. Nothing is further from the truth. Faculty today face unprecedented pedagogical challenges associated with the number of academically underprepared students entering college who are balancing more life roles and responsibilities than previous generations of students. "Such scenarios often cause a disjuncture between faculty expectations and student capabilities" (Moe & Murphy, 2011, p. 58). You must have a general understanding of who your students are if either you or they are to achieve the mutual goal of preparing them to be future health professionals.

Gateley, C. A. *Clinical Practice to Academia: A Guide for New and Aspiring Health Professions Faculty* (pp. 121-141). © 2021 Taylor & Francis Group.

The nature of our students—their academic preparation, aspirations, and cognitive development—affects our choices of what and how to teach.... Knowing both who your students are and how their minds learn is the starting point for teaching at its best (Nilson, 2010, p. 3).

Characteristics of Today's College Students

Each year over 20 million students enroll at approximately 4,600 degree-granting institutions across the United States (Thelin, 2017). We think of the traditional American college experience as attending an institution full time for 4 years immediately after high school (Stansbury, 2017). That traditional experience is rare for most college students today. Today's college student population is diverse and includes more first-generation college students, students of color, and students from low socioeconomic backgrounds than ever before (Bill & Melinda Gates Foundation, 2017, 2018). Only 55% of students are under 21 years of age, and 40% are 25 years old or older (Bill & Melinda Gates Foundation, 2018). Approximately 40% of students attend a community college, and the majority of those students cannot afford to attend full time (Mellow, 2017). Students also face more obligations beyond the classroom than their predecessors did. "The priority students affix to their education is too often usurped by increasingly demanding and time-intensive life priorities such as work, family, or emotional/psychological needs" (Crone & MacKay, 2007, p. 18).

Most students are employed (Bill & Melinda Gates Foundation, 2018), with 40% of students working 30 or more hours per week (Mellow, 2017). Additionally, 28% of students are parents (Bill & Melinda Gates Foundation, 2018). Unfortunately, half of the students who begin some level of postsecondary study leave before earning a certificate or degree (Bill & Melinda Gates Foundation, 2017).

> Many of these students don't have the support they need to balance demanding schedules and competing priorities. One of the biggest obstacles they face is an educational system designed to serve students who arrive straight from high school, live on campus, and study full-time. That is at least part of the reason why half of students who begin a college education don't reach graduation. (Bill & Melinda Gates Foundation, 2018, para. 2)

UNDERSTANDING DIFFERENT
GENERATIONS OF STUDENTS

Although age is only one of many factors that determine an individual's attitude about and approach to higher education and work, it is helpful to understand some general background and characteristics of different generations to understand why they think and behave the way they do. "Generations, much like cultures, have their own attitudes, beliefs, social norms, and behaviors that define them . . . ," and ". . . as every new generation emerges, it is subjected to a certain level of disdain from older generations" (Seemiller & Grace, 2016, p. 1). You are likely to encounter many of these diverse generations not only among your students but also among your colleagues and the clients your students will eventually serve. It is important for both you and your students to recognize and understand these differences in behaviors, perceptions, and expectations among generations and how those differences affect the college experience and professional practice. In the following sections, I briefly introduce concepts related to traditionalists, baby boomers, and Generation X. I will focus more of my attention on the two most recent generations, millennials/ Generation Me and Generation Z/iGen because they are the students you are most likely to encounter in the classroom. My intent is not to propagate stereotypes about particular generations but rather to help you better understand general trends identified by social and educational researchers. For every characteristic attributed to a particular generation, you will find exceptions among your students, but you will also start to recognize the behaviors described in the following sections in your students, colleagues, and clients.

Traditionalists

Traditionalists, also referred to as *Veterans* or the *Silent Generation*, were born between the 1920s and 1940s and experienced the Great Depression, World War II, and the Cold War. This generation has been described as disciplined, patriotic, loyal, and respectful of authority (McCready, 2011; Oblinger, 2003). They tend to be thrifty and hardworking, and they are used to adhering to rules.

Baby Boomers

Baby boomers were born between the 1940s and the 1960s. They grew up in a healthy, post–World War II economy and saw hard work as the way to a successful future (Seemiller & Grace, 2016). In the majority of families, their fathers worked, and their mothers stayed home to raise the children. Their life experiences included the civil rights movement, the space race, the Vietnam War, Watergate, Woodstock, and the assassinations of John F. Kennedy and Martin Luther King Jr. Defining characteristics of the baby boomer generation include a competitive nature, an optimistic outlook, a focus on personal growth and fulfillment, questioning of authority, and community involvement (Glass, 2007; Twenge, Campbell, Hoffman, & Lance, 2010).

Generation X

Generation Xers were born from the mid-1960s to approximately 1980 and witnessed world events including the fall of the Berlin Wall, expansion of mass media, the AIDS epidemic, the *Challenger* explosion, and the advent of the internet. They are described as skeptical, self-reliant, independent, and entrepreneurial (Glass, 2007; Oblinger, 2003). It was common for this generation to have both parents working; thus, they became known as "latchkey kids" because they were home alone after school (Seemiller & Grace, 2016). They saw increased rates of divorce among their parents and their own generation, and they experienced the hardships of the 2008 economic recession.

If you have Generation Xers in your classroom, they are likely juggling work and family responsibilities and want to complete their degree programs as quickly as possible. They may be returning to college for a second career, or they may be pursuing higher education for the first time. They bring with them life experience and perspectives that can enhance classroom discussions and learning for all students. However, they often have little tolerance for the antics of their less serious younger classmates and may feel left out if the majority of students in your class are millennials and Generation Z. Students in this generation are intrinsically motivated and appreciate knowing why something is important to learn (Campbell, 2016).

Millennials

Millennials, also known as Generation Y and Generation Next, were born from approximately 1980 to 2000. Please note that the birth year for the upper range of this generation varies by source. For example, Tai (2014) includes individuals born through 2004 in the millennial generation. This generation experienced Desert Storm, the Oklahoma City bombing, the Columbine shooting, and the September 11th terrorist attacks. Having grown up with personal computers, the internet, and cell phones, they are described as techno-savvy and multitasking (McCready, 2011). Howe and Strauss (2000, 2003) described them as "The Next Great Generation" and identified the following seven core traits that characterized this generation:

1. Special: For their entire lives, millennials were told that they were special. "Since birth, older generations have instilled in them the sense that they are central to their parents' sense of purpose and vital to the wellbeing of the nation" (Howe & Nadler, 2010, p. 111). Parents of millennials often remain very involved in their children's lives throughout the college years, and millennial students expect structure and frequent positive feedback in the classroom (Howe & Strauss, 2003). In the workplace, millennials want an expedited application and hiring process, a welcoming work environment, and mentoring programs (Howe & Nadler, 2010).

2. Sheltered: Millennials have grown up very protected by their parents, and they want to continue feeling safe when they get to college (Howe & Strauss, 2003). In addition to campus security, that feeling of safety also includes expectations of high grades for participation and effort rather than academic performance, and they and/or their parents are quick to complain about grades or threaten

litigation when things do not go their way. In the workplace, sheltered millennials expect a work–life balance, good insurance plans, and flexible scheduling (Howe & Nadler, 2010).

3. Confident: Millennials experienced K–12 education that was highly focused on self-esteem (Howe & Strauss, 2003). Millennial college students like to know the rules, and they will follow them and work very hard. They recognize safety in numbers and tend to avoid risk taking. Their confidence results in lofty career expectations and an expectation for positive feedback and frequent recognition to reinforce their confidence in the work setting (Howe & Nadler, 2010).

4. Team oriented: The millennial generation grew up in an environment that emphasized teamwork in everything from *Barney & Friends* videos to sports to volunteering (Howe & Strauss, 2003). They are not hung up on issues like race or ethnicity that divided previous generations, and they do not like participating in debates or peer critiques. They demonstrate a collaborative and interactive learning style. Millennials appreciate employers that provide group recognition for performance, engage in social networking, and showcase diversity (Howe & Nadler, 2010).

5. Conventional: Millennials exhibit more traditional lifestyles and attitudes than their parents did (Howe & Strauss, 2003). They seek out big brands in everything from clothing to college because they want to fit in, not stand out. They are very concerned about grades and rules, and they want organization and clear expectations in the college classroom because they want to know exactly how to succeed. In the workplace, they may need to have clearly defined rules about issues that older generations take for granted, such as appropriate attire and communication skills. They also want clearly defined expectations from their employers about what is expected of them in terms of work performance (Howe & Nadler, 2010).

6. Pressured: Millennials have experienced increased homework in earlier grades, longer class periods, and pressure from parents for high academic performance in order to get into the best colleges (Howe & Strauss, 2003). Upon entering college, they may have difficulty achieving a healthy balance between work and play, thus leading to burnout and sleep deficit disorders. Because of their pressured lives, some millennial college students may be more prone to cheating to maintain high grades. Having experienced collaborative pedagogy throughout their K–12 education, they also may have a hard time understanding what constitutes plagiarism or cheating, so these issues must be very clearly defined for them by higher education institutions. In terms of employment, millennials often feel pressured to choose a career in their teens and then carry out a well-defined strategy for achieving their career goals (Howe & Nadler, 2010). They seek employers who provide ongoing continuing education and career development as well as excellent salary and benefits.

7. Achieving: Millennials have been described as "the most all-around capable teen generation this nation, and perhaps the world, has ever seen" (Howe & Strauss, 2003, p. 123). In addition to high academic achievement, they also excel in extracurricular activities and community service. Despite getting good grades in high school, many millennials arrive at college underprepared in speaking,

writing, and numeracy. In college, they prefer subjects in which progress can be objectively measured, such as math and science, over fields that are more subjective in nature, such as the arts and humanities. They want to use technology and they expect straightforward grading policies. Because they have been so focused on academic achievement and multitasking their entire lives, millennials sometimes lack professional skills, such as phone and email etiquette and knowing what is or is not appropriate work attire. However, given clear guidelines, smaller benchmarks, and frequent performance reviews, millennials are certain to live up to employer expectations (Howe & Nadler, 2010).

A Different View of Millennials

In contrast to the relatively positive view of millennials described by Howe and Strauss (2000, 2003), academic researcher Jean Twenge presented a very different view of this generation in her 2006 book *Generation Me: Why Today's Young Americans are More Confident, Assertive, Entitled–and More Miserable Than Ever Before*. She described a sheltered generation raised by helicopter parents who scheduled every minute of their children's lives and swooped in to fix any problem that arose. She also critiqued teacher training programs at the K–12 level that focused more on providing a positive atmosphere than correcting mistakes. Twenge explained this resulted in a generation of college students who cannot accept criticism and who feel entitled to good grades simply for showing up to class because they grew up in an environment where everyone got a ribbon or trophy just for participation. Generation Me students may expect professors to reschedule exams that interfere with their vacation plans, give them an A for trying hard, and provide extra credit so they can get an A when they do not meet the original course expectations for that grade (Twenge, 2009).

Because they have been told repeatedly that they can be or do anything they want, Generation Me often has unrealistic expectations about entry into competitive degree programs, such as those in the health profession (Twenge, 2006). These high expectations carry on into the workplace where "jobs are no longer just jobs; they are lifestyle options" (Barlow, as cited in Twenge, 2006, p. 80). As a result, many employers complain that Generation Me employees have outlandish expectations for high salaries, flexible schedules, and speedy promotions.

Because Generation Me expects more yet finds success harder to attain, they have an increased incidence of depression and anxiety (Twenge, 2006). They are also more likely to argue with professors over grades or employers over what they view to be unfair treatment in the workplace. "As more GenMe'ers reach adulthood over the next few years, there will be a full-scale collision between their high expectations and the unfortunate realities of modern life" (Twenge, 2006, p. 213).

Generation Z

Like all generations, the date range assigned to Generation Z varies greatly by source and overlaps somewhat with the prior generation. Seemiller and Grace (2016) and Beall (2017) described Generation Z as individuals born from 1995 to 2010. Twenge (2017) used a range of 1995 to 2012. However, the U.S. Chamber of Commerce Foundation (2012) considers individuals born in or after 2000 part of Generation Z. Regardless of which generation they fall into, these students are headed to your classrooms over the next several years. Seemiller and Grace (2016) explained that Generation Z will make up one third of the U.S. population by 2020, and they will continue entering the workforce until 2032. Generation Z is the most racially diverse generation the United States has ever seen. In fact, they are likely the last generation in which White people make up the majority. They are also very close to their parents, with most Generation Zers reporting daily communication.

Beall (2017) described the following eight key differences between Generation Z and their predecessors, the millennials:

1. Less focused: Generation Z has grown up in a world of continuous updates and quick information processing, so their attention spans are likely to be significantly lower than millennials.

2. Better multitaskers: "Though Gen Z can be less focused than their Millennial counterparts, in school they will create documents on their school computer, do research on their phone or tablet, while taking notes on a notepad, then finish in front of the TV with a laptop, while face-timing with a friend.... Gen Z can quickly and efficiently shift between work and play, with multiple distractions going on in the background" (Beall, 2017, para. 4).

3. Less worried about bargains: Millennials reached or were approaching adulthood at the time of the 2008 recession. They were likely to clip coupons and click on online advertisements and reviews before making purchases. Individuals in Generation Z are overall less concerned with bargains.

4. Early starters: Rather than opting for the traditional route of higher education straight out of high school, many Generation Zers are creating new pathways for their future by going straight into the workforce and pursuing online education and other ways of educating themselves.

5. More entrepreneurial: Generation Z desires more independent work environments, and 72% of Generation Z teens have aspirations of starting their own business.

6. Higher expectations: "Generation Z was born into a world overrun with technology. What was taken [by Millennials] as amazing and inspiring inventions, are now taken as a given for teens" (Beall, 2017, para. 8).

7. Bigger on individuality: Although millennials were concerned about fitting it, Generation Zers are more comfortable with being unique and putting their individuality on display through social media.

8. More global: Generation Z has always had fingertip access to news, advertising, and social connections around the world. They are used to diversity and are more comfortable thinking about global issues and interacting with others beyond their own country.

Another View of the Current Generation

As you likely have noticed in reading this chapter, each generation is studied by numerous researchers who each form different interpretations and explanations of generational characteristics and behaviors. Just as Twenge (2006) coined her own term, *Generation Me*, for millennials, she also has her own moniker for this generation. Twenge (2017) argued that Generation Z is not an appropriate label for this generation because Generation Y never caught on as the popular label for the previous generation. She prefers the term *iGen*, referring to technology that this generation has always known. "The Internet was commercialized in 1995," and "according to a fall 2015 marketing survey, two out of every three US teens owned an iPhone, about as complete a market saturation as possible for a product" (Twenge, 2017, p. 2).

Twenge (2017) presented her research on the current generation in a recent book entitled *iGen: Why Today's Super-Connected Kids Are Growing Up Less Rebellious, More Tolerant, Less Happy–and Completely Underprepared for Adulthood*. It is a quick and fascinating read presenting easy to understand explanations of educational and social research on this generation. I highly recommend it to anyone considering a transition into academia, but for now I will briefly summarize Twenge's key points about iGen. She suggests that the "i" in iGen stands for the following characteristics:

- In no hurry–growing up slowly: You likely have seen or heard the hashtag #adulting on some form of social media in recent years. iGen is less interested in achieving particular milestones that were commonplace for previous generations. For example, iGen'ers are more likely to be accompanied by their parents to the mall or movies well into their teen years, less likely to get a driver's license at age 16, and less likely to have had a part-time job in high school where they would have learned responsibility, work ethic, and professionalism. "The entire developmental trajectory, from childhood to adolescence to adulthood, has slowed" (Twenge, 2017, p. 41).

- Internet–online time: This generation spends hours and hours online every day posting, viewing, and interacting with peers through Instagram, Snapchat, BuzzFeed, Twitter, YouTube, video chat, and online gaming. "Smartphones are unlike any other previous form of media, infiltrating nearly every minute of our lives, even when we are unconscious with sleep" (Twenge, 2017, p. 50).

- In person no more: "iGen'ers spend less time interacting with their peers face-to-face than any previous generation" (Twenge, 2017, p. 71). They are likely to have experienced, witnessed, or participated in cyberbullying. They also get far less practice with in-person social skills compared to previous generations. As a result, they may struggle with making new friends and interviewing for college or jobs.

- Insecure–the new mental health crisis: The high screen time described earlier has been linked to less overall happiness. iGen'ers are constantly comparing themselves to others through social media and experience a high level of "FOMO" or fear of missing out. They see pictures of friends at an event they weren't invited to. They see the new clothes or car their friend just got or the exciting vacation that someone else is on. iGen'ers often experience feelings of inadequacy when they see others' social media profiles and posts. A lack of "likes" or responses to their own posts and texts can lead to anxiety and sadness. They also experience insecurity and anxiety because of the increased pressure for high academic performance. Because they spend hours in bed looking at their phones, iGen'ers experience greater levels of sleep deprivation, which exacerbates their mental health issues.
- Irreligious: iGen'ers are less likely than any previous generation in the United States to attend church services or even claim affiliation with a particular religion.
- Insulated–not intrinsic: Having been supervised and protected every moment of their lives, iGen'ers expect physical and emotional safety to continue when they reach college. They demonstrate less risky behaviors than their previous counterparts, making them less likely to engage in physical altercations, risky sexual behavior, and drinking. Growing up with parents who intervened and handled any unpleasant situation for them, they expect campus administrators and faculty to do the same. They may demand "safe spaces," which are places "where people can go to protect themselves from ideas they find offensive" (Twenge, 2017, p. 154). This topic has been all over the news and social media in recent years as incidents of campus unrest continue to rise. Students participating in activism for social change are met with derogatory remarks from peers, politicians, and the general public calling them "snowflakes" and "crybabies" (Yagoda, 2016). I cannot do justice to discussing this topic in this brief section. If you are planning a transition to academia, I suggest you explore websites and recent news stories from the institutions you are considering. You are likely to find that this remains a hot topic, and you should have an idea of the issues that exist on a particular campus and how faculty and administrators have addressed those issues.

  In terms of being less intrinsic, Twenge (2017) explained that iGen'ers are more interested in extrinsic life goals, such as money, fame, and image. They see the primary purpose of college as preparing them for a career and are less concerned with higher education as a way of learning for the sake of learning.
- Income insecurity: Coupled with the focus on future careers, iGen students are worried about attaining good-paying jobs to pay off student loans. They are less confident and more realistic than millennials in terms of their expectations for educational and job attainment. They also desire a good work–life balance.
- Indefinite: sex, marriage, and children: iGen'ers are waiting longer to get married and have children. The average age of marriage has increased by 7 years over the last 5 decades, and fewer individuals are getting married at all (Twenge, 2017). Although there is still somewhat of a "hookup culture" with apps like Tinder and Grindr, Twenge reports that, compared to previous generations, fewer iGen'ers are having sex, fewer are in committed relationships, and fewer prioritize marriage and family.

- Inclusive: iGen'ers have grown up with diversity. "From LGBT identities to gender to race, iGen'ers expect equality and are often surprised, even shocked, to still encounter prejudice" (Twenge, 2017, p. 227). Interestingly, "iGen'ers get to college, where they earnestly strive for equality but are so afraid of offending one another that they still don't talk about race" (Twenge, 2017, p. 258).
- Independent: If you pay any attention whatsoever to news or social media, you know that the animosity between political parties has reached unprecedented levels. Yet, iGen'ers are less likely to affiliate themselves with a particular political party and often describe themselves as independent in their political views (Twenge, 2017).

TEACHING MILLENNIALS AND GENERATION Z

I grew up smack dab in the middle of Generation X, and I am the proud parent of two daughters born in 1998 and 1999. Depending on the source, they fall at the end of the millennial generation or the beginning of Generation Z. I personally am guilty of exactly what Twenge (2006) described in raising my children. From preschool through high school, our lives revolved around getting them to Girl Scouts, church youth group activities, birthday parties, playdates, and a ridiculous number of sports practices and games, and we loved every minute of it. As Twenge described, my daughters received medals and trophies for everything in which they participated, regardless of performance. Figure 9-1 shows all the medals my daughter received by age 13 for participation in various clubs, school events, and sports. Figure 9-2 shows the medals she actually earned based on individual or team performance against peers.

I also have spent much of my academic career teaching millennials and iGen'ers. I have experienced my fair share of some of the challenging behaviors described in these generations. However, I long ago came to the realization that, as a college instructor, I could spend my time complaining about students and hating my job, or I could learn to better understand my students and figure out ways to help them achieve success in the classroom while enjoying my role as an educator. I recognized that I could adapt my instructional strategies without compromising my standards for student performance.

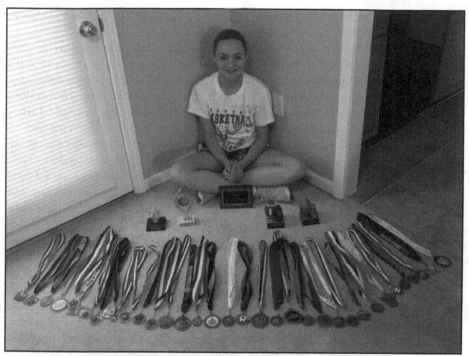

Figure 9-1. Total "awards" received by age 13, most for participation only.

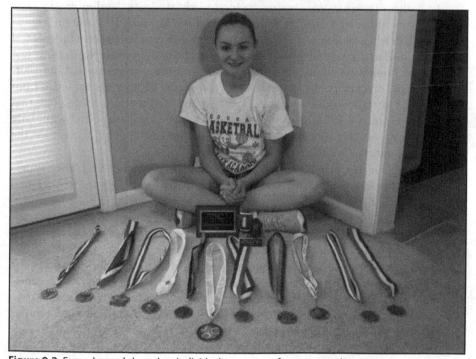

Figure 9-2. Earned awards based on individual or team performance against peers.

Price (as cited in Tai, 2014) identified the following key themes for educating this generation of students:

- Relevance: Students want to know why it is important to learn what you are trying to teach them. In health professions education, many topics and skills are obviously related to the students' future careers as health care professionals. However, sometimes instructors have to help students make those connections by relating the subject matter to current issues and events. For example, I teach a course for occupational therapy students entitled "Leadership, Management, and Policy." I have yet to meet a student who entered our professional program because he or she wanted to become a manager or policymaker. Students typically enroll in our program because they want to pursue clinical careers. I have to help students understand how policy can affect the documentation and reimbursement for clients in various settings and how leaders will monitor their productivity and conduct performance reviews.

- Rationale: Students are more likely to put forth good effort when they understand the reasoning behind material and policies presented to them. At the beginning of every course, and throughout the semester, I explain to students the accreditation standards covered in my course and how the course content relates to other courses and their overall curriculum within our program. I also explain to students any changes I have made based on previous course recommendations and why I have particular policies related to attendance, timeliness of assignments, and professional behavior.

- Relaxed: Students tend to perform better in less formal learning environments. As health care educators, we are trying to help students develop professional behaviors along with clinical skills; however, it is possible to maintain professionalism while facilitating a relaxed classroom environment where students feel more comfortable participating and asking questions. For example, in those last awkward moments before class starts when I am ready to get started but waiting for the exact start of class time, I sometimes play a funny animal video from YouTube or walk around the classroom and say, "Tell me something good that happened this week?" One of my colleagues starts each class period with daily trivia from her day-by-day calendar and provides a little prize or treat for the student who answers correctly.

- Rapport: Students desire a strong connection with their educators. They appreciate feeling like their instructors care about them and their performance in a class. Today's college students are more hesitant to speak up in class for fear of being wrong. "It takes more reassurance and trust to get them to actively participate in class" (Twenge, 2017, p. 307). As I encounter each new cohort of students, I share a bit of personal and professional information about myself including a few PowerPoint (Microsoft) slides with pictures of my family and pets and a list of all the health care jobs I have had in my career. I also try to learn a little something about each student. For example, I have had students complete one-page questionnaires with questions about their hometown, other life roles, campus and community activities, and so on. I have also had students write a one-page autobiography or create an introductory PowerPoint slide to share with the class.

These ideas work well for smaller classes, but there are other things you can do in larger lecture courses. Consider having students create table tents with their names by folding a piece of paper in thirds. This allows you to call students by name when you ask questions during class. After each exam, send group emails to all the students who did well congratulating them on their performance, and to all the students who did poorly send suggestions on improving their performance on the next exam or assignment.

- Research-based methods: Decades ago, lecture-based teaching was the primary means of instruction. Today's students appreciate learning in a variety of ways. Chapter 11 provides several ideas of instructional strategies. Depending on the topic you are presenting, consider a mix of other active learning strategies. For example, if I want students to learn about credentialing and licensure requirements, they will learn much more from a guided online exploration of the websites for the credentialing agencies and state licensure boards than from me lecturing to them about the requirement. I also include videos, small group discussions, hands-on labs, and other activities that present the material in a more effective way than lecturing.

Sanchez (2016) agreed that today's college students prefer experiential, collaborative learning to lecture. They are used to a constant stream of information at their fingertips and often do not exhibit attention spans adequate for retaining information presented through lectures and dense reading. Twenge (2016) suggested "short, readable passages interspersed with activities" to help students absorb material. Students also appreciate instant gratification, even if that gratification is simply knowing if they were correct or incorrect in a response. Many college instructors now use student response systems, or "clickers," for in-class quizzes or simply to check students' understanding of the material presented. These devices look similar to a remote control, and student responses are tallied by an electronic device the instructor has at the front of the classroom. Students can instantly see how their responses compare to those of their classmates.

Many college instructors implement a "flipped classroom" strategy in which students are expected to complete readings or watch recorded lectures before class, and class time is spent in applied and experiential learning. It has been my experience that many students are somewhat resistant to this method the first time they encounter it. I once had a student write on a course evaluation that "I felt like I was teaching myself. I thought that was your job." What that particular student did not recognize was the time and effort I had put into selecting the right readings and videos to help students prepare for the activities we would be doing in class. My colleagues and I have also observed that most students eventually see the benefit to this approach. Talbot (2018) reported similar findings across flipped classroom research, explaining that "these benefits only tend to sink in over time. Students often have highly negative views on flipped learning when it is first introduced; and some students persist with those views throughout the course" (para. 15).

"Truly great teachers have always tried to teach students how to teach themselves" (Scott, 2007, p. 215).

MINORITY STUDENTS

"College is often an exciting and unique place to be for students and faculty alike … but for minorities, colleges can also be inaccessible and hostile places" (Lynch, 2016, para. 1-3). Many minority students are first-generation college students, and they and their families may be unfamiliar with how to navigate the college environment. Additionally, many minority students graduate from high school academically unprepared for college as a result of long-standing socioeconomic disparities. "It seems that all of the energy that goes into trying to 'change' minority students who enter the classroom would be better spent adjusting teaching methods to ones of inclusion" (Lynch, 2016, para. 12). Folk (2018) also advocated moving away from a deficit perspective of minority students and instead using the funds of knowledge that students bring to the classroom through their identities and lived experiences. Can you provide small group discussion prompts that allow students to share something about their backgrounds that ties to the topic of the day? Can you create assignments that encourage students to reflect on how personal experiences from their own lives will impact their careers as future health care professionals?

You need to be cautious about singling out minority students. "'Singling out a student' occurs when a faculty member or student calls on a fellow student to represent a group or educate the rest of the class about a group to which the student belongs" (Portman et al., n.d., p. 1). Doing so creates the assumption that this particular student knows and shares the opinions and experiences of everyone who shares the same identity. We often think of "minority" as only meaning racial and ethnic minorities, but we also need to consider that we may have students in our classrooms who are a minority in terms of gender identity, sexual orientation, religious background, ability level, and countless other differences.

The University of Denver Center for Multicultural Excellence conducted a student-led workshop in 2008 during the Annual Diversity Summit. Workshop participants shared numerous stories of times when they had been singled out by a classroom professor or targeted by classmates without any intervention from the instructor. These incidents occur on every college campus, whether intentional or not, and can negatively impact minority students' sense of belonging and willingness to engage in the classroom. A few other students shared examples of times when professors facilitated positive conversations about minority issues that helped minority students feel more included and helped other classmates to better understand minority perspectives. If you want to facilitate a more inclusive learning experience, look for campus resources and events that will make you more aware of how what you do as an instructor affects the minority students in your classes. Make an intentional effort to address minority issues in your course, particularly as they relate to your health care profession.

"In thinking about the phenomenon of singling students out, the following are some questions for faculty members to consider in addressing this issue:

- What is the climate for diversity like in your classroom?
- How might you inadvertently be singling out students?
- Are some of your students targeting other students?
- What will you do in situations where you or other students are tempted to or actually do single out students?
- What can you do to make your classroom more inclusive for gay, lesbian, bisexual, transgender, intersex, and queer students; students of color; international students; women; men; students from different religious backgrounds; students with disabilities; and students from other salient groups of the campus community?
- Do students representing different backgrounds feel 'safe' in your classroom?
- Are the exercises, assignments, examples, and syllabus inclusive?
- As with all aspects of our teaching, a little extra forethought and in-the-moment attention can help us avoid/prevent the issue of singling out students in our classrooms and contribute to an inclusive classroom that maximizes learning for everyone." (Portman et al., n.d., pp. 5-6)

What Do Students Want in an Instructor?

Years ago at the Wakonse Conference on College Teaching, I learned a technique called "Mutual Expectations" (2010). On the first day of class, I ask students to write down what characteristics they appreciate in an instructor. Depending on the size of the class, it also works well to have students discuss this in small groups and turn in one paper per group. I then collect the papers and make a list or PowerPoint that I review during the next class period to discuss how I plan to meet certain expectations and why I may not be able to meet other expectations. I have been doing this activity for years, and student responses are much the same every year. Although this list is not comprehensive, the most common student comments are that they appreciate an instructor who does the following:

- Is enthusiastic and knowledgeable about the subject
- Encourages questions and discussion
- Uses a variety of teaching methods
- Provides real-life examples that relate to course content
- Provides feedback in a timely manner
- Responds to emails in a timely manner
- Understands that students have lives beyond one particular class

I believe those all seem like reasonable expectations for a college instructor. However, regarding email response time, I make it clear to my students that I will respond to emails Monday through Friday during work hours, but if they email me in the evening or on a weekend, my response time may be somewhat delayed because that time is for my family. As long as I make this policy clear at the beginning of the semester, students are typically satisfied. I also make exceptions to my own policy if I know students have an exam, project, or assignment coming up that will generate several questions. Depending on your setting, the expectations may differ, particularly if you are teaching an online course. This is a question you should ask your department chair and colleagues.

One of my colleagues recently introduced me to the Ask Three Before Me strategy (Bankston, 2018; G. Pifer, personal communication, June 4, 2018), which encourages students to solve problems independently by making attempts to answer questions on their own rather than immediately emailing the instructor regarding things like due dates, assignment expectations, class attendance policies, and other information that likely is already available somewhere. For example, students can refer to the syllabus, look on the online learning management system course page (e.g., Canvas, Blackboard), or ask a classmate. This strategy significantly reduces the number of student emails requesting information that you likely have already communicated in one or more ways.

RISING MENTAL HEALTH ISSUES

High school and college students are dealing with mental health issues in unprecedented numbers (James, 2017). College counselors are seeing a sharp rise in students with anxiety, depression, and more serious psychiatric disorders, including self-injury and suicidal thoughts. Novotney (2014) reported that one-third of college students had difficulty functioning in the past 12 months because of depression, and nearly one-half had experienced overwhelming anxiety in the past year. Many mental health conditions begin before 24 years of age, but students may have difficulty talking with their families about these issues.

Although it is beyond your role as an instructor to provide counseling services, it is your responsibility to be familiar with the campus resources available to students and to guide students toward those services when appropriate. Most campuses have some type of counseling center or crisis hotline. I have had many students come to my office and tell me about a wide variety of problems, including relationship issues, illness or death of a loved one, long-standing anxiety issues, and substance abuse problems, all of which may impact their attendance or performance within the classroom. In many instances, students just want me to know their situation, and they seem to be handing it well on their own. Other students need more support than I can provide in my role as an instructor and academic advisor, and in those cases, I refer them to professional counseling. Many students are hesitant to seek out services at the campus counseling center on their own. On multiple occasions, particularly when I believe the student is in a crisis situation, I have called the counseling center with them and even walked them across campus to the initial appointment. Unfortunately, despite the rising numbers of mental health issues among college students, 32% of campus counseling centers have a waiting list at some point during the academic year (Novotney, 2014).

STUDENTS WITH DISABILITIES

Students who have various types of disabilities that affect their educational experience are eligible for accommodations within the higher education settings. Most campuses have a disability center or some office within student services that helps students establish an accommodation plan. As the course instructor, you will receive communication from the student regarding accommodations for your particular course. You should work directly with the student and disability center to determine how best to implement the accommodations within your course. Common accommodations may include the following:

- Alternative textbook formats: Students may have textbooks that have been converted to a digital format or may use a text-to-speech software that reads the book to them. Unless you are having students read a textbook during class, this accommodation likely would not affect you as the instructor.
- Classroom and lab assistants: Students with physical disabilities may have a classroom or lab assistant present to help them lift and manipulate objects. Students with visual deficits may have an assistant to describe objects and visual course content to them.
- Accessible tables, chairs, and rooms: Students who use wheelchairs or other mobility devices may require special seating. The disability center arranges for the equipment to be placed in your classroom, but you may need to remind other students to leave those spaces open for the students who need them.
- Exam access: This is one of the most common accommodations that I have experienced with my students. Many students require reduced-distraction or distraction-free environments and/or additional time for exams. In some situations, I have been able to provide this accommodation myself by scheduling a time for the student to take the exam in a private room. When I have multiple students in the same course with this type of accommodation, my program simply does not have the space or staff to proctor multiple students on an individual basis. In those situations, I send the exam to the disability center, and the students schedule a time with the center to take the exam under the conditions that I specify. For example, I have the option as the instructor to specify that students take the exam at the same time or same day as their peers, and I can specify whether or not students may use notes during the exam.
- Communication access: Students with hearing impairments may have a sign language interpreter or assistive listening device to help them understand your lecture and classroom discussion. You may be asked to wear a microphone to assist in this process.

- Note-taking assistance: At my institution, when students qualify for note-taking assistance, the disability center asks me to send out an email to the class asking for volunteers to take notes and provide them to the disability center; the center then provides the notes to the student with the accommodation.
- Flexible attendance: This accommodation can be a bit disconcerting to faculty, particularly if you have strict attendance policies in your course. I have been advised by our campus disability center that this accommodation is a not a free pass to miss an unlimited number of days. Rather, each instructor can determine what is reasonable for a particular course. For example, if you typically allow one or two absences without penalty, you may allow a student with a flexible attendance accommodation three or four absences. You may also require the student to do additional outside work each time he or she misses class.

Students with accommodations are not required to disclose to their instructors the reason for their accommodations. At the same time, instructors are not expected to alter the essential functions of their courses. The best strategy is to remind all students at the beginning of the semester to communicate with you as soon as possible about accommodations they may have and then meet directly with the student to develop a plan that addresses the student's needs while meeting your course expectations. When questions or issues arise, the disability center staff are available to help students and faculty discuss and implement accommodations. It is important to remember that accommodations are meant to level the playing field for students with a disability rather than giving them an advantage over other students.

CONCLUSION

Hopefully, this chapter helped you understand some of the characteristics of contemporary college students and some of the issues you may encounter as you help them become members of your health profession. Each semester you will encounter new challenges with students. I strongly recommend that you make an effort to get to know your students and understand their backgrounds and expectations. Through a collaborative effort, you and your students can all have a positive teaching-learning process.

LEARNING ACTIVITIES

1. Think about what kind of student you were when you went through your professional program. How old were you? What was your approach to learning? Were you focused on always getting an A or just happy that you passed a class? Did you always put in maximum effort to ensure that you learned everything you could from a reading or assignment, or did you do the bare minimum that was required? Did you prefer learning on an individual basis or with a group of students? What other roles did you have when you were in college? Were you balancing school, work, extracurricular activities, and/or family responsibilities? Which type of student did you tend to spend time with? If you are currently enrolled in a course, discuss these topics with your classmates.

2. Think about a college instructor who you really enjoyed having as a teacher? What did he or she do that you really liked? Now think about an instructor that you did not like? What was different about his or her approach to teaching? What are your expectations for an instructor? Which characteristics do you want to exhibit in your teaching?

3. Think about people you know who fall into the various generational categories of veterans, baby boomers, Generation X, millennials, and iGen. Which characteristics described in this chapter do you see in them? Are there differences in their behavior compared to the characteristics that researchers attribute to their generation? This is a great topic for class discussion or an online discussion board.

4. Explore the demographic information for the student population of an institution where you currently work or hope to work in the future. Are there a large number of nontraditional college students? How diverse is the student population in terms of race and ethnicity? Are there any organizations or services on campus for specific minority groups?

5. Search recent literature on teaching the current generation of college students. This is a common topic in books, academic journals, and other publications. Beyond the information provided in this chapter, what additional insights and suggestions did you locate regarding teaching this generation?

6. Explore your institution's campus resources related to equity, diversity, and inclusion. Are there resources available to help you as an instructor make your classroom more inclusive?

7. Explore your institution's resources related to disability services. How do students become eligible for disability accommodations? Are there resources for instructors? Discuss with classmates any concerns you may have about implementing accommodations in a course that you may teach in the future.

8. What counseling or other mental health services are available on your campus? How do students access these services? As an instructor, how can you assist students in gaining access to these services? Are there any resources for faculty and staff in addressing student mental health concerns?

REFERENCES

Bankston, K. (2018). Ask three before me. BetterLesson. Retrieved from https://betterlesson .com/strategy/69/ask-three-before-me

Beall, G. (2017, November 6). 8 key differences between Gen Z and Millennials. *Huffington Post.* Retrieved from https://huffingtonpost.com https://www.huffingtonpost.com/george-beall/8-key-differences-between_b_12814200.html

Bill & Melinda Gates Foundation. (2017). The changing face of U.S. higher education: How new students are coping. *The Washington Post.* Retrieved from http://www.washingtonpost.com/sf /brand-connect/gates/the-changing-face-of-us-higher-education

Bill & Melinda Gates Foundation. (2018). Today's college students. Retrieved from https:// postsecondary.gatesfoundation.org/what-were-learning/todays-college-students/

Campbell, S. (2016). 9 things to consider when starting to work with adult learners. CAEL. Retrieved from https://www.cael.org/blog/9-things-to-consider-when-starting-to-work-with-adult-learners

Crone, I., & MacKay, K. (2007). Motivating today's college students. *Peer Review, 9*(1), 18. Retrieved from https://www.aacu.org/publications-research/periodicals/motivating-todays-college-students

Folk, A. L. (2018). Drawing on students' funds of knowledge: Using identity and lived experience to join the conversation in research assignments. *Journal of Information Literacy, 12*(2), 44-59. doi: 10.11645/12.2.2468

Glass, A. (2007). Understanding generational differences for competitive success. *Industrial and Commercial Training, 39*(2), 98-103. doi:10.1108/00197850710732424

Howe, N., & Nadler, R. (2010). *Millennials in the workplace: Human resource strategies for a new generation.* Great Falls, VA: LifeCourse Associates.

Howe, N., & Strauss, W. (2000). *Millennials rising: The next great generation.* New York, NY: Vintage Books.

Howe, N., & Strauss, W. (2003). *Millennials go to college: Strategies for a new generation on campus.* Washington, DC: American Association of Collegiate Registrars.

James, S. D. (2017, June 28). Mental health problems rising among college students. NBC News. Retrieved from https://www.nbcnews.com/feature/college-game-plan/mental-health-problems-rising-among-college-students-n777286

Lynch, M. (2016, December 26). How to provide minorities with a richer college experience. *The Edvocate.* Retrieved from https://www.theedadvocate.org/how-to-provide-minorities -with-a-richer-college-experience

McCready, V. (2011). Generational issues in supervision and administration. *The ASHA Leader, 16*(5), 12-15.

McGraw Hill Education. (2017). Five lessons about today's college students that we can apply in 2017. Retrieved from https://www.mheducation.com/blog/thought-leadership/college-student-lessons-to-apply-2017.html

Mellow, G. O. (2017, August 28). The biggest misconception about today's college students. *The New York Times.* Retrieved from https://www.nytimes.com/2017/08/28/opinion/community-college-misconception.html

Merisotis, J. (2017, July 14). Not who you think: The truth about today's college students. *The Washington Post.* Retrieved from https://www.washingtonpost.com/news/grade-point/wp/2017/ 07/14/not-who-you-think-the-truth-about-todays-college-students/?utm_term=.98cf43b1b2c7

Moe, A. M., & Murphy, L. M. (2011). Being a new faculty. In E. Lenning, S. Brightman, & S. Caringella (Eds.), *A guide to surviving a career in academia: Navigating the rites of passage.* New York, NY: Routledge.

Mutual Expectations. (2010, May). Session presented at 2010 Wakonse Conference on College Teaching, Shelby, MI.

Nilson, L. B. (2010). *Teaching at its best: A research-based resource for college instructors.* San Francisco, CA: Jossey-Bass.

Northern Illinois University. (n.d.). Millennials: Our newest generation in higher education. Faculty Development and Instructional Design Center. Retrieved from https://www.niu.edu/facdev/_pdf/ guide/students/millennials_our_newest_generation_in_higher_education.pdf

Novotney, A. (2014). Students under pressure: College and university counseling centers are examining how nest to serve the growing number of students seeking their services. *Monitor on Psychology, 45*(8), 36. Retrieved from http://www.apa.org/monitor/2014/09/cover-pressure.aspx

Oblinger, D. (2003). Boomers, Gen-Xers, and Millennials: Understanding the new students. *EDUCAUSE Review, 38*(4), 36-47.

Portman, J., Ogaz, J., Turner, C., Valdez, V., CdeBaca, C., Devereaux, V., ... Trevino, J. (n.d.). *Singled out: Student stories of the diversity challenges and opportunities in the classroom.* Retrieved from http://otl.du.edu/wp-content/uploads/2013/03/SingledOutInClassroom-DUCME.pdf

Sanchez, S. (2016). The millenial learners: Changing the way we learn and teach. Inside Higher Ed. Retrieved from https://www.insidehighered.com/blogs/university-venus/millennial-learners

Scott, A. F. (2007). Why I teach by discussion. In A. L. Deneef & C. D. Goodwin (Eds.), *The academic's handbook* (3rd ed., pp. 212-216). Durham, NC: Duke University Press.

Seemiller, C., & Grace, M. (2016). *Generation Z goes to college.* San Francisco, CA: Jossey-Bass.

Stansbury, M. (2017, July 8). 3 big ways today's college students are different from just a decade ago. *eCampusNews.* Retrieved from https://www.ecampusnews.com/campus-administration/college-students-different/

Tai, W. A. (2014, April 16). *Millenial learners.* Retrieved from https://teachingcommons.stanford.edu/teaching-talk/millennial-learners

Talbot, R. (2018, March 1). *What does the research say about flipped learning?* Retrieved from http://rtalbert.org/what-does-the-research-say/

Thelin, J. R. (2017). *American higher education: Issues and institutions.* New York, NY: Routledge.

Twenge, J. M. (2006). *Generation Me: Why today's young Americans are more confident, assertive, entitled–and more miserable than ever before.* New York, NY: Atria Paperback.

Twenge, J. M. (2009). Generational changes and their impact in the classroom: Generation Me. *Medical Education, 43*(5), 398-405. doi:10.1111/j.1365-2923.2009.03310.x.

Twenge, J. M. (2016). Generation Me: Understanding and teaching today's students. Pearson. Retrieved from https://www.pearsoned.com/generation-me-understanding-and-teaching-todays-students/

Twenge, J. M. (2017). *iGen: Why today's super-connected kids are growing up less rebellious, more tolerant, less happy–and completely unprepared for adulthood.* New York, NY: ATRIA Books.

Twenge, J. M., Campbell, S. M., Hoffman, B. J., & Lance, C. E. (2010). Generational differences in work values: Leisure and extrinsic values increasing, social and intrinsic values decreasing. *Journal of Management, 36*(5), 1117-1142. doi:10.1177/014920630935226.

U.S. Chamber of Commerce Foundation. (2012). *The Millennial Generation research review.* Retrieved from https://www.uschamberfoundation.org/reports/millennial-generation-research-review

Yagoda, B. (2016, December 4). Who you calling Snowflake? *The Chronicle of Higher Education.* Retrieved from https://www.chronicle.com/blogs/linguafranca/2016/12/04/who-you-calling-snowflake/

10

Conceptual Foundations of Teaching and Learning

Like many of the topics in this book, there are entire texts dedicated to conceptual foundations of teaching and learning. It is beyond the scope of this chapter and this book to provide a comprehensive overview that gives due diligence to the collective work of scholars who have written about teaching and learning. Rather, my intent in this chapter is to present a brief overview of a few resources that have helped me in my role as a college educator. In clinical practice, we expect students and practitioners to seek out resources to help them stay up to date with new discoveries and to engage in evidence-based practice. Health professions education is constantly evolving, and we as educators should always be looking for new ideas to improve our instructional strategies and enhance student learning. My hope is that the ideas presented in this chapter will serve as a foundation for your own professional development as you transition from practitioner to educator.

"Teaching and learning are among the most complex activities in which human beings engage, and neither is fully understood" (Scott, 2007, p. 212).

PEDAGOGY AND ANDRAGOGY

Pedagogy is used broadly to refer to "the study and theory of the methods and principles of teaching" (Collins English Dictionary, n.d.). However, looking more closely at the root of the word, pedagogy refers to the teaching of children, just as pediatrics refers to a branch of medicine dealing with children (Association of College and Research Libraries, n.d.). In contrast, *andragogy* focuses on the teaching of adult

Gateley, C. A. *Clinical Practice to Academia: A Guide for New and Aspiring Health Professions Faculty* (pp. 143-156). © 2021 Taylor & Francis Group.

TABLE 10-1

PEDAGOGY VERSUS ANDRAGOGY

	PEDAGOGY	ANDRAGOGY
LEARNER SELF-CONCEPT	Learners are dependent on the instructor for what will be taught and how it will be evaluated.	Learners are self-directed, responsible for their own learning, and evaluate their own learning.
PRIOR EXPERIENCES OF THE LEARNER	Learners have little past experience to build on and serve as a learning resource.	Learners use past life experiences to make connections as they learn new concepts and skills.
READINESS TO LEARN	Learners are told what they need to learn, with a focus on mastery in order to progress to the next level.	Learners understand the value of education and are serious and focused about learning.
ORIENTATION TO LEARNING	Learning is subject centered, and learners focus on memorizing content.	Learning is problem centered and focused on addressing real-life and work situations.
MOTIVATION TO LEARN	Learners are extrinsically motivated by rewards and punishments for academic performance.	Learners are internally motivated and satisfied with the feeling that they have learned something.
NEED TO KNOW	Learners accept the authority of the instructor in determining what they need to learn.	Learners need to understand why something is relevant for them to learn.

Adapted from Knowles, M. S., Holton III, E. F., & Swanson, R. A. (2005). *The adult learner: The definitive classic in adult education and human resource development* (6th ed.). Burlington, MA: Elsevier.

learners (Knowles, Holton, & Swanson, 2005). Table 10-1 summarizes the differences between pedagogy and andragogy. However, the question is which approach should you follow as a college instructor. My advice is that you need to understand both approaches. Depending on your setting, degree level, and student population, you may have learners who are still very much used to and desire a pedagogical approach to teaching and learning. On the other hand, if your program has a large percentage of adult learners who are pursuing a degree in their late 20s, 30s, and beyond, they may benefit from, and be more open to, approaches based on the andragogical model.

In my own experience, you are likely to have a wide variety of learners in your classroom. I like to view my role as helping them along a continuum from pedagogy to andragogy. Many students enter our competitive admission program with histories of exceptional academic performance, and they are focused on earning an A in every course. I tell them repeatedly, course after course, that the most important letters for their future are "OTR/L," which stands for occupational therapist registered and licensed. In other words, the grades for a particular assignment or course do not matter as much as them learning what they need to know to pass the board exam and become an occupational therapist. Most of them gradually make the transition to self-directed, intrinsically motivated learners. Some never do. Being aware of the differences between pedagogy and andragogy helps me understand why students approach the learning process in very different ways and that I need to be flexible in how I design learning experiences for a diverse group of learners.

LEARNER-CENTERED TEACHING

In recent years, health professions education programs have shifted away from teacher-centered pedagogy, in which the instructor is at the center of learning, toward a model of learner-centered pedagogy, also known as student-centered learning (Patel-Junankar, 2018). Weimer (2002) described the following five characteristics of learner-centered teaching:

1. Balance of power: Students are motivated and empowered by having some control over the learning process
2. Function of content: Instructors move away from covering content and instead focus on using content to help students develop skills such as problem solving and the ability to evaluate evidence.
3. Role of the teacher: Instructors engage students by designing meaningful learning experiences and serving as a guide and facilitator as students encounter the content rather than having it provided to them by the instructor.
4. Responsibility for learning: Students experience a shift in thinking about learning as something that they are required to do toward an understanding that they want to show up and engage in learning because it is important to their present and future goals.
5. Purpose and process of evaluation: Although instructors still award final grades, learners are engaged in self- and peer evaluation throughout the learning process as they reflect on what and how they are learning.

Bloom's Taxonomy: Original and Revised

In 1956, educational psychologist Benjamin Bloom and several colleagues published the *Taxonomy of Educational Objectives*, which became popularly known across K–12 and higher education as *Bloom's Taxonomy* (Armstrong, 2017; Bloom & Krathwohl, 1956). The original taxonomy contained the following categories, or objectives of learning, progressing from simple to complex in terms of the cognitive abilities expected of students:

- Knowledge: Recall of ideas
- Comprehension: Understanding of material without transferring it to other situations
- Application: Applying principles to specific situations
- Analysis: Breaking down complex ideas into small parts and understanding their relationship
- Synthesis: Bringing together ideas from multiple sources to form new, integrated ideas
- Evaluation: Making judgments of ideas and methods based on evidence and observations

In 2001, a group of cognitive psychologists, educational researchers and theorists, and assessment specialists published a revision of Bloom's original work with the new title *A Taxonomy for Learning, Teaching, and Assessing: A Revision of Bloom's Taxonomy of Educational Objectives: Complete Edition* (Anderson & Krathwohl, 2001). "This title draws attention away from the somewhat static notion of 'educational objectives' (in Bloom's original title) and points to a more dynamic conception of classification" (Armstrong, 2017, para. 9). The authors of the revised taxonomy used the following verbs, rather than nouns, to describe the cognitive processes involved in each category and subcategory of the taxonomy:

- Remember: Recognizing, recalling
- Understand: Interpreting, exemplifying, classifying, summarizing, inferring, comparing, explaining
- Apply: Executing, implementing
- Analyze: Differentiating, organizing, attributing
- Evaluate: Checking, critiquing
- Create: Generating, planning, producing

In the revised taxonomy, knowledge is still the basis of the six cognitive processes listed, but the authors describe four different types of knowledge used in cognition:

1. Factual knowledge: Terminology, details, elements
2. Conceptual knowledge: Classifications and categories; principles and generalizations; theories, models, and structures
3. Procedural knowledge: Subject-specific skills, algorithms, techniques, and methods and the criteria for determining when to use them
4. Metacognitive knowledge: Strategic knowledge, knowledge about cognitive tasks, and self-knowledge

How are these taxonomies useful to a novice health professions educator? They help you think about the purpose of a course, or even a particular class session, and determine what you want your students to accomplish as a result of your teaching. A simple online search of "Bloom's Taxonomy verbs" or "revised Bloom's Taxonomy action words" will give you dozens of ideas for measurable actions that you can use as you write course or session learning objectives. If you teach in a health professions program overseen by an accrediting entity within your profession, be sure that your learning objectives match the accreditation standards required for your particular degree program.

FINK'S TAXONOMY OF SIGNIFICANT LEARNING

In 2003, L. Dee Fink, a renowned professional and international consultant in higher education, introduced a new taxonomy that went beyond the cognitive domain of Bloom's taxonomy and its subsequent revision. Fink (2013) defined learning in terms of change.

> For learning to occur, there has to be some kind of change in the learner. No change, no learning. And significant learning requires that there be some kind of lasting change that is important in terms of the learner's life. (p. 34)

As opposed to the hierarchical nature of Bloom's taxonomy and the taxonomy for teaching, learning, and assessment, Fink's taxonomy of significant learning recognized the interactive and synergistic relationships of the following types of learning (Fink, 2013, pp. 34-36):

- Foundational knowledge: Understanding and remembering ideas and information
- Application: Skills; managing projects; and engaging in critical, creative, and practical thinking
- Integration: Connecting ideas, learning experiences, and realms of life
- Human dimension: Learning about oneself and others
- Caring: Developing new feelings, interests, and values
- Learning how to learn: Inquiring about a subject, becoming a better student, and becoming a self-directed learner

Fink (2013) recognized that students may achieve many types of learning simultaneously and that achievement in one type of learning is likely to enhance achievement in other types of learning. Fink suggested two major implications of his taxonomy for college instructors: (a) learning outcomes for a course must go beyond mastery of content and (b) using a combination of learning objectives creates synergistic effects to enhance student achievement of significant learning.

As with Bloom's taxonomy and a taxonomy for teaching, learning, and assessment, instructors can locate numerous online resources for use of Fink's taxonomy of significant learning to help develop learning objectives for each type of learning.

Many novice, and even experienced, college teachers approach course design by simply organizing a list of topics into the schedule of the course (Fink, 2013). Although quick and easy, this approach often results in a lecture-laden course with little attention to the quality of student learning. Other college instructors approach course design with a list of activities to make the course more interesting and to engage students in active learning. Although this approach reduces the emphasis on lecturing, it still has little focus on learning. Fink (2013) suggested a learning-centered approach that he called "integrated course design" (p. 68).

In the integrated course design approach, Fink (2013) explained that instructors have information that needs to be gathered and decisions that need to be made regarding the connected components of learning goals, feedback and assessment, and teaching and learning activities. Fink (2013) introduced a 12-step process of integrated course design divided into the following 3 phases:

Initial Phase: Building Strong Primary Components of the Course

1. Size up the situational factors, such as the number of students, type of classroom, place of your course in the overall curriculum, nature of the subject, student and instructor characteristics, and pedagogical challenges.
2. Determine the learning goals or learning outcomes for the course, being sure to go beyond foundational knowledge to include other types of learning including application, integration, human dimension, caring, and learning how to learn.
3. Formulate feedback and assessment procedures that help you know if students have achieved the learning outcomes you identified in Step 2.
4. Select teaching and learning activities that engage students in active learning through experiences and reflection on what and how one is learning.
5. Make sure that the primary components identified in Steps 2, 3, and 4 are all integrated by identifying assessment procedures and learning activities for each learning outcome you have identified for your course. Identify the resources needed to support each learning activity.

Intermediate Phase: Assembling the Components Into a Dynamic, Coherent Whole

6. Create a thematic structure for the course by identifying approximately four to seven major ideas or topics and arrange them in an appropriate sequence in which ideas build on one another.

7. Select or create a teaching strategy that will effectively accomplish the learning outcomes you have identified. Fink (2013) distinguished between a teaching technique, which is a specific activity, such as lecturing or using small group discussions, and a teaching strategy, which "is a particular combination of learning activities, arranged in a particular sequence ... that work together synergistically and build a high level of student energy that can be applied to the task of learning" (p. 144).

8. Integrate the course structure and instructional strategies to create an overall scheme of learning activities that students will encounter both in and outside of class. This process will help you lay out a week-by-week schedule of activities for the duration of your course.

Final Phase: Finish Important Details

9. Develop a grading system that reflects the full range of learning goals and activities and reflects the importance of each activity. Fink reminded instructors that not everything has to be graded.

10. Review your plan and think about what might go wrong. Have you considered all the situational factors? Do you have a good mix of learning outcomes and appropriate assessment methods? Do students have adequate time and resources to accomplish everything you are expecting of them?

11. Develop your course syllabus to let students know your plan for the course, including instructor information, course goals, structure and sequence, required readings, grading procedures, and other course policies.

12. Plan an evaluation of the course and your teaching performance. Think beyond the standard student end-of-course bubble sheet assessments that your campus likely requires. Consider midterm assessments from students or classroom observations and feedback from a peer faculty member.

If you find Fink's (2013) approach intriguing for your own use, please know that my very brief summary is not a sufficient resource to embark on the time-intensive process of integrated course design. Fink provides detailed explanations and numerous examples for each step of the approach in his book *Creating Significant Learning Experiences, Revised and Updated: An Integrating Approach to Designing College Courses*. Numerous online and in-person workshops on this strategy are also available.

FACILITATING SEVEN WAYS OF LEARNING

Davis and Arend (2013) introduced a framework for matching intended learning outcomes with distinct ways of learning and instructional strategies. Based on decades of literature on teaching and learning, they identified seven ways of learning that college instructors may attempt to facilitate in their classes. Like Fink (2013), Davis and Arend recommended that instructors first identify their intended learning outcomes, which "are not a list of topics to cover. They are what the learner is supposed to get from or do with the subject" (2013, p. 33). Davis and Arend explained that there are three levels of learning objectives:

1. Global objectives: Written at the program or college level
2. Educational objectives: Written at the course level
3. Instructional objectives: Written for an individual class session, lesson, or unit

Davis and Arend's (2013) framework focused on the instructional objective level. In other words, what do you want your students to know or be able to do after a particular class, session, or unit? The authors listed three precautions in selecting appropriate ways of learning:

1. Do not randomly select and use several ways of learning in hopes that at least one thing will work for your students.
2. Do not select a way of learning based on students' preferred learning styles. The way of learning should be based on the desired learning outcome.
3. Do not select a way of learning based on your own comfort level.

The sections that follow include a brief discussion about each learning outcome, the associated way of learning, and common instructional methods that align with each way of learning. As with other approaches described in this chapter, if you are interested in implementing Davis and Arend's approach, be sure to review their book *Facilitating Seven Ways of Learning: A Resource for More Purposeful, Effective, and Enjoyable College Teaching* for a more thorough understanding of how to facilitate each type of learning.

Building Skills: Behavioral Learning

This category of learning outcomes includes "physical and procedural skills where accuracy, precision, and efficiency are important" (Davis & Arend, 2013, p. 45). Examples include inserting a nasogastric tube, demonstrating correct hand movements for sign language, operating ultrasound equipment, or using a goniometer to measure a client's range of motion. These skills typically involve a set of actions that require practice for mastery. Based on behavioral learning theory, common instructional methods to help students master skills include providing students with modeling and hands-on opportunities to practice the exercise, task, or procedure and giving students step-by-step directions with specific feedback so they can improve their performance. Instructors may need to perform a task analysis to break down the desired skill into substeps.

Acquiring Knowledge: Cognitive Learning

In this category of intended student learning outcomes, instructors want their students to acquire "basic information, concepts, and terminology in a discipline or field of study" (Davis & Arend, 2013, p. 71). Examples include identifying the muscles required for a certain movement, understanding the terminology associated with a particular profession's conceptual framework, or recalling which functions each area of the brain controls. Cognitive learning theory provides a good basis for helping students acquire knowledge with its focus on attention, information processing, and memory. Instructors may assign readings, give lectures with PowerPoint or Prezi (Prezi Inc), or have students watch videos or other multimedia presentations that help them learn new material. Davis and Arend explained that instructors should help students know what to focus on and help students with making meaning of new material as they compare it to existing knowledge.

Developing Critical, Creative, and Dialogic Thinking: Learning Through Inquiry

This category of learning outcomes involves improved thinking and reasoning processes, such as critiquing information, evaluating evidence, appreciating what others think, producing new ideas, and being aware of one's own thinking (Davis & Arend, 2013). Examples include evaluating the pros and cons of a particular treatment approach for a given diagnosis, creating a new method or piece of adaptive equipment to compensate for a client's deficits, and developing empathy for opposing arguments and viewpoints. Students improve their thinking and reasoning processes as they learn through inquiry. Instructors can facilitate inquiry through student discussion with a partner or small group using open-ended questions that invite narrative responses. Davis and Arend (2013) explained that facilitating learning through inquiry is something that must be embedded throughout a course, not just a single class session:

> Developing thinking skills takes time … critical, creative, and dialogic thinking should be part of nearly every class in colleges and universities. Students need to be informed of the purpose of inquiry and learn to get better at thinking under expert guidance over time. (p. 133)

Davis and Arend also emphasized the need for instructors to create a safe environment for students to participate in inquiry and thinking without feeling judged for their thoughts.

Cultivating Problem-Solving and Decision-Making Abilities: Learning With Mental Models

This category of learning outcomes involves solving problems, making decisions, and finding solutions. Students may need to define problems and organize their knowledge into systematic strategies as they weigh various options and choose a solution. Using mental models as a way of learning, students create a mental image of the situation and make predictions about the outcome of various solutions, picturing each step as they think through the problem. The common instructional methods used by teachers trying to facilitate this type of learning are problems, case studies, lab activities, and projects. Students often work together in small teams to solve problems and make decisions. The role of the instructor is to provide enough background information for students to tackle the problem and then help them sort out irrelevant information and to "keep the focus on the process and steps rather that the final solution or decision" (Davis & Arend, 2013, p. 173).

Exploring Attitudes, Feelings, and Perspectives: Learning Through Groups and Teams

Instructors may identify student learning outcomes that include developing empathy; understanding multiple perspectives; or changing attitudes, opinions, or beliefs. These learning outcomes are best facilitated through group activities and team projects. Davis and Arend (2013) identified the following prominent approaches to team-based learning:

- Cooperative learning: Students work together harmoniously to find an answer.
- Collaborative learning: Students work together as part of a learning community where dissent and disagreement are encouraged for deeper learning.
- Team-based learning: This approach typically involves a combination of in- and out-of-class activities, and less time is spent on facilitating the group process skills.
- Problem-based learning: Students work together to address complex, unstructured cases. Instructors serve as tutors whose role is to facilitate the group process and help students focus on the most relevant information to the case.

Instructors may have to help students work through common problems such as conflict, apathy, lack of adequate contribution by a group member, or groupthink, which occurs when groups prematurely reach a conclusion because no one wants to disagree and risk conflict.

Practicing Professional Judgment: Learning Through Virtual Realities

This type of learning outcome involves the student demonstrating "sound judgment and appropriate professional action in complex, context-dependent situations" (Davis & Arend, 2013, p. 213). Students need the opportunity to practice professional judgment in safe, simulated environments to gain confidence and competence before exposure to real situations that may result in damage, expense, or threat to well-being or life. Based on psychodrama, sociodrama, and gaming theory, the common instructional methods to facilitate this type of learning are simulations, games, dramatic scenarios, and role-playing that help students apply existing knowledge to novel situations. In the health professions, instructors may use strategies such as role-play scenarios with classmates, video cases, standardized patients, or high-tech simulated models. Instructors must be prepared to observe and intervene if needed to help students complete the simulation experience. Debriefing after the experience is important to help students reflect on what went well, identify areas for future improvement, and process any emotional reactions they may have had to the experience.

Reflecting on Experience: Experiential Learning

Based on the theory that students construct knowledge through experience and reflection, this type of learning typically involves internships, service learning, study abroad, and other real-life experiences. Students have the opportunity to apply previous learning to new situations and develop an awareness of their own identities and how they influence others. An important component of experiential learning is reflection in action, in which students "must think about what they are doing while they are doing it, and it is in this way they learn from experience" (Schön, as cited in Davis & Arend, 2013, p. 248). Instructors must match students with settings that meet their educational needs, help students define responsibilities and learning goals, and guide ongoing reflection to facilitate meaning-making from the students' experiences.

CURRICULUM DESIGN AND CURRICULUM MAPPING

The concepts of curriculum design and curriculum mapping are closely related to the teaching and learning approaches presented in this chapter. Think back to when you first began college. Did you think about how each course was part of an overarching plan for your particular degree? Or, did you simply take whichever courses your academic advisor told you were required? Unbeknownst to most students, higher education institutions and the individual programs that comprise them have curriculum designs that serve as plans for educational goals and how the courses will be structured and sequenced to meet those goals (West, Loftin, & Snyder, 2018). In health professions educational programs, your accrediting agency may require that your program have a written and graphic representation of your curriculum design and how it relates to accreditation standards. Prideaux (as cited in West et al., 2018) explained that curriculum design involves the following four elements:

1. Content
2. Teaching and learning strategies
3. Assessment processes
4. Curriculum evaluation

Faculty and administrators may use curricular mapping to create a visual representation of the curriculum and to increase collaboration among faculty within and across departments (Uchiyama, 2008). Curriculum mapping is as follows:

> A process used to identify when, where, and how content is addressed across the curriculum in an effort to recognize gaps and redundancies; to ensure that content is introduced, reinforced, and assessed; to guarantee that instruction and assessment are aligned to what students are expected to learn; and to promote self-study and critical analysis. (Calloway, 2018, p. 35)

Curricular mapping may involve a simple matrix using a Word or Excel (Microsoft) document that shows the relationship between courses and overall program goals. More recently, educators and administrators have turned to curriculum mapping software that provides users and reviewers with various ways of looking at both the big picture and the details of particular courses and strategies in teaching, learning, and assessment. During a recent accreditation review, my department relied on a matrix to demonstrate to reviewers how we addressed various accreditation standards and program goals through individual coursework and overall curriculum design. Our campus has a new center for teaching and learning, and the director recently asked faculty and administrators to explore a curriculum mapping system that can be used in departments across the institution. Although I was initially reluctant to commit the time to learning a complex new system when we already had an effective strategy that helped us achieve reaccreditation, after more thought, I volunteered to participate in a trial of the program to see if it may benefit our department with future curriculum revision and program accreditation efforts.

If you are pursuing a faculty position, ask your department chair and faculty colleagues about your program's curriculum design and whether curriculum mapping is something that your program has done in the past. If you have the opportunity to serve on a committee involved in these processes, it is a great opportunity to gain a better understanding about how each piece of the curriculum relates to the larger goals of the program and institution.

CONCLUSION

Reading through these various approaches to teaching and learning may seem overwhelming to a new college educator. Each time I learn about a new strategy, I think to myself, "Why wasn't I doing this before?!" Then I realize that the important thing is that I am willing to learn about and implement new approaches to improve my teaching. Throughout your academic career, you should never think that you know everything you need to know about teaching. There is always something new you can learn and changes you can make.

LEARNING ACTIVITIES

1. Review the differences between pedagogy and andragogy. Think about your own educational experiences. Which approach did your college instructors use? How did you respond? Were there changes over time in how you approached learning? Why? How can you use these insights to plan learning experiences for your students?

2. Reflect on your college academic experience. Can you identify examples of when instructors used learner-centered approaches?

3. Perform an online search to locate action words associated with each category of *A Taxonomy for Learning, Teaching, and Assessing*. Write educational objectives appropriate for your discipline for each category of the taxonomy.

4. Perform an online search to locate action words associated with each category of Fink's taxonomy of significant learning. Write learning objectives appropriate for your discipline for each category of the taxonomy.

5. Locate a copy of *Facilitating Seven Ways of Learning: A Resource for More Purposeful, Effective, and Enjoyable College Teaching*. Develop instructional objectives relevant for your profession for each way of learning and identify appropriate learning activities to address each instructional objective.

6. Find out if your department has a curriculum design or curriculum philosophy. Some academic programs have these posted on their websites. You may have to ask a faculty member or department chair for the document. Explore any accreditation standards for your profession related to curriculum design. Look for scholarly articles in your discipline about curriculum design. Search for software products relevant to curriculum design in the health professions.

REFERENCES

Anderson, L. W., & Krathwohl, D. R. (Eds.). (2001). *A taxonomy for learning, teaching and assessing: A revision of Bloom's Taxonomy of educational objectives: Complete edition.* New York, NY: Longman.

Armstrong, P. (2017). *Bloom's Taxonomy.* Vanderbilt University Center for Teaching. Retrieved from https://cft.vanderbilt.edu/guides-sub-pages/blooms-taxonomy/

Association of College and Research Libraries. (n.d.). *Keeping up with andragogy.* Retrieved from http://www.ala.org/acrl/publications/keeping_up_with/andragogy

Bloom, B. S., & Krathwohl, D. R. (1956). *Taxonomy of educational objectives: The classification of educational goals, by a committee of college and university examiners. Handbook 1: Cognitive domain.* New York, NY: Longman.

Calloway, C. A. (2018). Curriculum mapping. In G. Kayingo & V. M. Hass (Eds.), *The health professions educator: A practical guide for new and established faculty* (pp. 35-44). New York, NY: Springer.

Collins English Dictionary. (n.d.). *Pedagogy.* Retrieved from https://www.collinsdictionary.com/dictionary/english/pedagogy

Davis J. R., & Arend, B. D. (2013). *Facilitating seven ways of learning: A resource for more purposeful, effective, and enjoyable college teaching.* Sterling, VA: Stylus.

Fink, L. D. (2013). *Creating significant learning experiences, revised and updated: An integrated approach to designing college courses.* San Francisco, CA: Jossey-Bass.

Knowles, M. S., Holton III, E. F., & Swanson, R. A. (2005). *The adult learner: The definitive classic in adult education and human resource development* (6th ed.). Burlington, MA: Elsevier.

Patel-Junankar, D. (2018). Learner-centered pedagogy: Teaching and learning in the 21st century. In G. Kayingo & V. M. Hass (Eds.), *The health professions educator: A practical guide for new and established faculty* (pp. 3-12). New York, NY: Springer Publishing Company.

Scott, A. F. (2007). Why I teach by discussion. In A. L. Deneef & C. D. Goodwin (Eds.), *The academic's handbook* (3rd ed., pp. 212-216). Durham, NC: Duke University Press.

Uchiyama, K. P. (2008). Curriculum mapping in higher education: A vehicle for collaboration. *Innovative Higher Education, 33*(4), 271-280.

West, H., Loftin, C. T., & Snyder, C. L. (2018). Curriculum design. In G. Kayingo & V. M. Hass (Eds.), *The health professions educator: A practical guide for new and established faculty* (pp. 13-24). New York, NY: Springer.

Weimer, M. (2002). *Learner-centered teaching: Five key changes to practice.* San Francisco, CA: Jossey-Bass.

11

Instructional Strategies for the Classroom and Clinic

Throughout this book, I have explained that many of the topics presented are too broad to be covered adequately in a single chapter and that you should explore other resources on topics of most importance to you. If I had to pick one chapter from this book in which it is most essential that you continue exploring new resources and implementing new strategies throughout your academic career, this is the one. Never be satisfied with your teaching! There are always improvements you can make to enhance student learning. I learn something new about teaching every semester, and I make an intentional effort to make changes in future courses. I challenge you to do the same.

In this chapter, I will begin with a few tips about course preparation and syllabus development. I will also introduce several instructional strategies commonly used in health professions education and briefly discuss assessment of student learning. I hope this chapter leaves you with more questions than answers, and I hope you use those questions to guide your future professional development efforts related to teaching.

COURSE PREPARATION

For the first few college courses I taught years ago, my course preparation consisted of reviewing recent syllabi for the course, making a few schedule changes, selecting some readings from a textbook, and coming up with a few learning activities, which, in retrospect, probably had little cohesion across the course. Flash forward 12 years, and I approach course preparation so much differently. I think about the purpose of the course and where it falls in our professional curriculum in relation to other courses. I think about the accreditation standards that are assigned to a particular

Gateley, C. A. *Clinical Practice to Academia:*
A Guide for New and Aspiring Health Professions Faculty
(pp. 157-174). © 2021 Taylor & Francis Group.

course and how I can address and assess each of those standards. I talk with other faculty who teach courses in the same semester to see if there are ways we can help students make connections between courses. I talk with faculty who taught my students in previous semesters so I understand what knowledge and skills they have when they reach my course. I talk with faculty who teach courses in future semesters so I understand what they expect students to know when they get to their courses. In recent years, my department has moved away from faculty doing course planning in isolation. Instead, we routinely review the curriculum and course content for each semester, collaborating with one another about schedules, textbooks, learning activities, and assessment strategies. We also co-teach many courses in our curriculum, which can be beneficial for both new and experienced faculty. As a new faculty member, you may have to seek out guidance with course preparation if you have not been assigned a particular faculty mentor. Ask to review the syllabi of other faculty. Ask faculty members to share advice about course preparation. Have other faculty review your course materials and provide feedback. This peer review process may even be required when you submit a dossier later on for promotion (see Chapter 7).

SYLLABUS DEVELOPMENT

Your department or institution may have a specific format or template that you need to use for your course syllabi. If no such template exists, ask for copies of syllabi from other faculty in your department to get you started. Although specific syllabus content may vary by institution, department, or course, here is a list of the basic information that, at minimum, you should include in a syllabus:

- Course title and number
- Department
- Semester
- Instructor and credentials
- Faculty contact information
- Office hours
- Course credits
- Course times and locations
- Course description
- Course objectives
- Grading scale
- Required textbooks and other course materials
- Attendance and professional behavior policies
- Course expectations
- Methods of assessment (e.g., exams, assignments, labs) and associated points
- Course schedule

You may also need to include campus-wide policies in your syllabus. For example, my campus has specific statements related to intellectual pluralism, the Americans with Disabilities Act, and making and distributing audio and video recordings of courses. If your program is accredited, the accrediting body may have specific requirements related to course syllabi, such as the inclusion of departmental mission and vision statements and accreditation standards.

DEVELOPMENT OF LEARNING ACTIVITIES AND ASSIGNMENTS

If you have not already done so, you may find it helpful to review Chapter 10 before you tackle the development of learning activities, assignments, exams, and other methods of assessing student learning. You have to think about the purpose of your course and the specific learning objectives affiliated with your course. What do you want your students to know or be able to do after they take your course? How can you best facilitate student learning to meet those expectations? This section contains several suggestions of instructional approaches that you may find useful in your courses.

Large Lecture Courses

I imagine most people reading this book have been part of a large lecture course at some point in their higher education. What constitutes large? That depends entirely on the subject matter and institution, but you get the picture—an auditorium or large classroom with rows of desks facing the front of the room, often with the instructor on a stage at a podium. Thinking back to your own experiences in such courses, what strategies did the instructor use to facilitate learning? Was the lecture the primary, or perhaps only, method of instruction? Did you ever skip that class? Why?

An online search for "tips for large lecture courses" will reveal dozens of articles and websites on this topic. If you are teaching a large lecture course, you need to explore those resources. A common theme is that you need to keep students engaged. Student attention tends to fade after about 20 minutes, so you need to stop every so often and do something new (Berkeley Center for Teaching and Learning, 2019). For example, show a video clip relevant to the class topic, relate course topics to a current news event and have students discuss in pairs or small groups, or administer a few clicker questions to assess student understanding. Ledlow (2001) suggested spending 5 to 10 minutes doing a think-pair-share or write-pair-share activity in which you pose a question and ask students to spend a few minutes thinking about or writing their responses, then sharing their responses with a partner, and finally calling on random students to share their ideas with the larger classroom to facilitate greater understanding of a topic.

Facilitating Classroom Engagement

Barkley (2010) suggested that "student engagement is a process and a product that is experienced on a continuum and results from the synergistic interaction between motivation and active learning" (p. 8). Motivated students want to learn, will seek information and understanding, and are a joy to teach. Unmotivated students will test the fortitude of even the most experienced faculty member.

> Just as a classroom filled with students who are genuinely motivated to learn can be teaching nirvana, it can be teaching hell trying to work with students who are apathetic, bored, or even hostile; or who are so compulsively obsessed with grades that they badger us incessantly to improve theirs on every assignment; or who seem deliberately to take on strategies that are self-defeating. (Barkley, 2010, p. 15)

Active learning is not as simple as forcing students to participate in small group activities or discussions (Barkley, 2010). The defining characteristics of active learning are active engagement of the mind, making connections between new information and past experiences, and reflection on both the product and the process of learning. Barkley (2010) suggested that faculty should strive to achieve the following three classroom conditions in order to promote synergy between motivation and active learning:

1. Create a sense of classroom community: Faculty need to facilitate collaborative activities that help students feel respected and valued as members of a learning community.

2. Help students work at their optimal level of challenge: "Somewhere between 'been there, done that' and 'dazed and confused' lies the optimal level of challenge that engages students.... Engaged learning occurs in the gap between a learner's current understanding and potential understanding" (Barkley, 2010, p. 48). Faculty need to analyze student performance and provide both summative and formative feedback. Summative feedback occurs at the end of a topic or unit, whereas formative feedback occurs throughout the learning process so students can make corrections and adjustments. Faculty should also encourage students to use metacognitive skills to monitor the effectiveness of their own learning.

3. Teach so that students learn holistically: Barkley (2010) explained that professors need to understand that learning is not a stand-alone cognitive function. The affective and psychomotor domains are also important to student learning. The affective domain refers to how students feel about the content they are learning and how they perceive the learning climate. "How students *feel* about what is happening in the classroom is critical to how they engage—or disengage—in the learning that teachers are trying to engender in the classroom" (Barkley, 2010, p. 35).

So, how do we, as educators, implement Barkley's (2010) recommended classroom conditions? I think this a never-ending goal for faculty. Each semester I try to implement at least one new strategy to create a sense of classroom community. Of course, the number of students in your classroom certainly impacts what you can do, but the following are a few suggestions:

- Have students use name tags to display their names on their desk. This makes it easier for you and other students to call each other by name during class discussion.
- During in-class small group discussions and activities, randomly assign students to groups to facilitate their engagement with students beyond the one or two classmates they tend to sit near.
- Have students fill out an index card with three facts about themselves. Throughout the first few weeks of the semester, or over the course of the semester for larger classes, read the cards aloud, and see if students can guess whose information you read. For some added fun, have students include one silly thing that others may not know about them.
- In small classes or academic programs where students move through as a cohort over several semesters, have each student select a photograph and write a brief "bio" to share with students and faculty. Compile these into a single electronic or hard-copy document for distribution.
- Place students into random small groups and explain to them that they have been put in these groups based on information you gathered from their various online profiles. Their task is to figure out what they have in common to have ended up in a group together. Give the groups 5 to 10 minutes to figure out commonalities before revealing that you really did not have time to stalk them online before class. Beyond serving as a way to help students understand that they can find common ground with almost anyone, it also reminds students that they should be cautious about how they present themselves on social media because someone unexpected might be looking at it. I was a participant in a similar activity at a professional development conference (University of Missouri Faculty Scholars, 2013). Years later, I still vividly remember that activity, and I often use it as an icebreaker early in the semester.

Faculty can use several different brief, low-stakes assessment measures throughout a course to gauge students' understanding of course concepts (Chew, as cited in Lang, 2012). For example, students can answer a question or complete a problem or short assignment and then compare with a neighbor or small group. Faculty can also use classroom response systems, or clickers, that allow students to respond anonymously to a posed question so that faculty and students see where their understanding falls in relation to the overall class. Faculty can also incorporate the use of "minute papers" in which they briefly write down responses to some variation of the following questions: (a) What did you learn today? and (b) What is still confusing? (Angelo & Cross, as cited in Lang, 2012).

Regarding holistic learning, I think it is important to have conversations with students about how they feel about my course in particular, their current overall educational experience, and life in general. Is it a particularly challenging semester? Are they feeling overwhelmed with the number of deadlines in a given week? Has a recent personal, local, or national event affected them in some way that may impact their academic performance? I may or may not make adjustments to my own course based on student feedback, but simply acknowledging that you understand that students are balancing multiple academic and personal obligations can go a long way toward creating a positive learning environment. If you use clickers in your classroom, a quick way to gauge where students are emotionally on any given day is to have them rate their current stress level on a scale from 0 to 10 using their clickers.

I also like to get students up and moving in the classroom whenever possible. Depending on your course and particular topic for the day, is there an activity you can plan in which students get hands-on practice with a particular skill, technique, or strategy? Can they brainstorm answers in small groups and write their suggestions on a whiteboard or flip chart? Rather than explaining something in a lecture format, can you have students works in pairs to locate the information online or in resources that you bring to class? For example, I keep many brochures that I receive in the mail for continuing education conferences. In one of my classes, I have students explore the brochures that are displayed around the classroom, select one event they would like to attend, and then work with a partner to develop a travel request that includes estimated travel expenses that they have looked up online. Another simple way to get students out of their seats and moving is to have a 5-minute break where students are expected to go find someone they have not yet met or engaged with, find out one thing about the person, and briefly discuss a topic from the day's class.

Barkley (2010) stressed the importance of faculty outreach on student engagement. "You have to reach out to students. You can't wait for them to reach out to you. The good students always have and always will reach out, but the struggling students don't know how to make the first move" (Barkley, 2010, p. 73). We often jump to the assumption that a struggling student simply is not trying or does not care. Ask the student to schedule a meeting with you and discuss his or her situation. You may discover that the student is balancing full-time work, family responsibilities, and academic deadlines. The student may be experiencing significant personal or family stress. Perhaps the student has a language or cultural barrier that is limiting his or her engagement and performance in your class. I often learn during these meetings that students do not know how to study in a rigorous health care curriculum. They are used to receiving As and Bs with minimal effort and inconsistent attendance in prerequisite coursework and are a bit shell-shocked with the significant increase in academic and professional behavior expectations when they enter a professional curriculum.

Problem-Based Learning

Problem-based learning (PBL) goes beyond using case studies as an instructional strategy. "PBL problems tend to be messier and fuzzier, and the course material alone cannot provide viable solutions" (Nilson, 2010, p. 187). Students must work in teams to conduct outside research and problem solve potential solutions. First introduced in medical school curricula in the 1960s, PBL has spread across health professions and other disciplines as an effective way to help students learn how to approach the uncertain challenges they will encounter in practice. A simple online search will reveal numerous variations on implementing PBL into a single course or across an entire curriculum. My goal here is to introduce you briefly to the concept. If it is a strategy that would be useful in your teaching, I strongly encourage you to explore additional resources and talk to other faculty who have used PBL in their own teaching. What follows in this section is a brief synthesis of just a few resources on PBL implementation.

Principles of Problem-Based Learning

PBL is characterized by students reviewing a complex case in small groups (approximately 4 to 10 depending on the overall course size), identifying learning needs, completing outside research to better understand the problem, sharing new knowledge with other group members, and using the new information to develop a plan of how best to approach assessment and intervention with the client. Instructors serve as tutors whose primary role is to monitor group process and provide facilitation only when a PBL group gets stuck and cannot unstick themselves, when groups stray too far from the relevant information in the case, or when group dynamics reach a point where student learning is compromised. Rather than providing answers, tutors ask guiding questions to help students explore possible answers on their own. Within each group, students may have assigned roles for a particular date or case. For example, one student may be assigned as the facilitator of group discussion, whereas another student is assigned as the scribe to record group comments as they review the case and share information. PBL is believed to be effective in helping health professions students meet the following learning objectives (Abdalla & Gaffar, 2011; Nilson, 2010):

- Collaborative teamwork and interpersonal skills
- Effective oral and written communication skills
- Tolerance for uncertainty
- Critical thinking and analysis
- Clinical reasoning skills
- Application of metacognitive strategies
- Self-directed learning behaviors
- Development of complex problem-solving and decision-making skills
- Increased sensitivity to patient needs

Problem-Based Learning Format

PBL is a multistep process that typically requires class periods of at least 2 hours each with adequate time in between class sessions for students to complete outside research. Following is one example of how PBL may be implemented into a course that meets on a weekly basis (Abdalla & Gaffar, 2011; Nilson 2010):

Week 1

- Introduce PBL as a teaching and learning strategy.
- Review roles of instructor (PBL tutor), group facilitator, and scribe.
- Set ground rules and expectations for preparation, participation, and group behavior.
- Introduce a mini-PBL case that can be completed in a single class period to help students understand what is likely a new method of learning for them.

Week 2

- Present students with a complex, ill-structured case that leaves them with more questions than answers. You may be able to locate cases specific to your discipline online or in textbooks. Alternatively, instructors often write their own cases based partially or entirely on actual client situations that they have encountered in practice, using caution to avoid breaking applicable patient privacy guidelines. You can present the case in stages to give students a little information at a time. For example, first give them an overview of how a client presented in the emergency department and intensive care unit. Then provide additional information about the client's presentation a few days or weeks later. Add in complicating family, socioeconomic, and other contextual factors.

- As they review the case, students identify the following:
  - What they know, or think they know
  - What they need to understand better: This is often where the tutor may need to provide a prompt or two to get students to consider relevant factors they may have overlooked or to skim over distracting information that is not essential to explore further.

- From the list of problems and subproblems identified in the previous step, students formulate learning objectives. In other words, what else do they need to learn before they can address the client's problems? They should brainstorm about where they might obtain the needed information. This is another step in which the tutor may have to provide some initial guidance or suggestion about how to seek out information. Students need to go beyond a simple Google search. Encourage them to explore discipline-specific databases of peer-reviewed journals. Remind them that libraries on your campus have resources that they may not be able to access online and librarians who are eager to help them find those resources. Suggest that they contact relevant professionals or agencies that may be able to provide additional information.

- Once learning objectives have been identified, students negotiate who is responsible for finding each piece of needed information and reporting back to the group during the next class period. Depending on the PBL group size and the number of learning objectives identified, students may need to combine and prioritize their learning objectives so the work is more evenly distributed.

Week 3

- After conducting research to address their assigned learning objectives, students report back to the group the information obtained and how it relates to the specific case at hand. As the PBL tutor, you can provide as much or as little guidance as you want in terms of how you want students to present their information to their classmates for learning and to you for grading. Options include, but are not limited to, informal discussion, formal paper with citations and references, presentation with or without visuals such as PowerPoint (Microsoft), or a brief handout summarizing the information. One area where students, especially those new to the PBL process, often struggle is in making adequate connections between the information they located and how it applies to the specific case they are reviewing. If other group members do not probe for this information, the tutor may have to facilitate group discussion, particularly if you think students are missing information that they need to move forward with addressing the case.
- As each student presents the information from his or her assigned learning objectives, students gain another piece of the puzzle. At the end of this class session, students should have a much better understanding of the client's complex situation and what steps to take next to address the client's needs. Each student's homework is to develop an intervention plan for the client.

Week 4

- Students return with a written intervention plan for the case study client. Depending on standard practice in your profession, this plan may include guiding theoretical principles, long-term goals, short-term goals, and specific intervention strategies to address each goal. As an added challenge, tutors may require students to role play one portion of their intervention plan with the tutor serving as the client. For a more realistic experience, you should simulate the physical and cognitive deficits of the client described in the case study, as well as the fluctuating motivation and willingness to participate that the students may encounter later on in practice. For example, if the student begins the intervention with "Hi, Mrs. Robertson. Are you ready to get out of bed?" you can respond with "No. I'm too tired today. Maybe tomorrow." This gives students the opportunity to think on their feet and modify their plan in a relatively safe environment.

Team-Based Learning

Originally developed in the late 1970s for growing enrollments in business education, faculty are now using team-based learning (TBL) in medical and health professions education (Wallace & Walker, 2018). Although PBL requires a faculty facilitator for each small group, TBL teams work in a classroom with one instructor with an emphasis on student collaboration, consistent preparation before class, and the ability to problem solve through discipline-specific structured activities. Teams typically consist of five to seven students, and TBL uses the following approach to teaching and learning:

- Before class, students acquire content knowledge through assigned readings, videos, or other structured activities.
- During class, students complete individual and team readiness assurance tests.
- After the readiness assurance test, faculty clarify major points, and students work with their teams on application-based exercises.
- Throughout the course, students complete self- and peer assessments of individual contributions and overall team performance.

Although TBL requires fewer faculty than PBL, it requires a considerable amount of time and effort from faculty who want to implement a TBL approach. Wallace and Walker (2018) recommend that faculty experience TBL firsthand as part of their training and preparation for implementing in their own courses. Additionally, students need to be prepared for TBL.

> It is not uncommon for students who expect passive forms of learning to express frustration with TBL. Students will be surprised by how much effort it takes to engage and problem solve. Advance planning and effective communication are key to successful implementation. Faculty must be explicit about why TBL was chosen for the class format and what students will gain from the experience. Students may need to be educated about how different learning strategies accomplish different levels of learning. (Wallace and Walker, 2018, pp. 75-76)

Flipped Classroom

Higher education scholars have been talking about flipped, or inverted, classrooms for 2 decades (Brame, 2013; Lage, Platt, & Treglia, 2000; Nichols, 2018). Using a flipped classroom approach, students gain exposure to new content before class via assigned readings, videos, case studies, recorded presentations, and other materials. Students then arrive to class prepared to process the material through learning activities that require analysis, synthesis, and problem solving while the instructor interacts with students and provides feedback (Brame, 2013). Instructors may implement strategies such as worksheets and quizzes to ensure that students come to class prepared, but the long-term goal is that students eventually recognize that adequate preparation before class contributes significantly to their learning.

Nichols (2018) cautioned that faculty who are intrigued by the concept of a flipped classroom need to start with small steps. Rather than trying to flip an entire course, which takes considerable time and planning, she recommended starting with one or two class periods. Take a look at your course as a whole "and identify its flippable moments; this will help you choose what, when, and how to flip" (Nichols, 2018, p. 81).

Lab Activities

In the health professions, we expect our students to demonstrate competence in entry-level skills. Hands-on laboratory experiences provide an excellent opportunity for students to practice and master those skills. For example, do your students need to know how to administer range of motion and manual muscle test screenings? Put them in pairs or small groups and have them practice on each other. If your students need to calculate chronological ages of children to administer and interpret standardized developmental assessments, create a worksheet that gives them numerous opportunities to practice calculation. If your students need to be able to take vital signs, plan a lab session that involves hands-on practice with blood pressure cuffs and stethoscopes. When you are planning lab activities, think about whether you also need to develop a lab checkout or other method of assessing student learning. Your accrediting body may require evidence of how you assess student competence with particular skills, and a simple checkout at the end of a lab session may meet some accreditation requirements.

Simulation

Health professions educators are increasingly using simulation as part of students' education. "Clinical simulation is an instructional design that substitutes real patient encounters with artificial models, live actors, or virtual-reality patients" (Walkup, Wishner, & Gardner, 2018, p. 131). One example of simulation is a model with accompanying software that allows students to practice venous and arterial access. Another example is an entire mannequin that simulates various patient symptoms. Such examples are very costly, but many programs find them well worth the investment in providing students with a low-risk option for training before working with real patients.

Another example of simulation in health professions education involves the use of standardized patients. "A standardized patient is someone who has been trained to portray, in a consistent, standardized manner, a patient in a medical situation" (University of Pittsburgh School of Medicine, 2016, para. 1). Standardized patients may be faculty, students in advanced cohorts, theater students, local professionals, or volunteers from the community. Standardized patients learn about a case and act out the patient's story as the student obtains the patient's history and conducts a physical examination. This method is beneficial in helping students develop competence and confidence with interviewing and communication skills as well as clinical assessment skills (Walkup et al., 2018).

ASSESSING STUDENT LEARNING

Just as there are numerous teaching and learning strategies that you may use as an instructor, there are a variety of ways to assess student learning. Meckel et al. (2018) summarized the complexity of learner assessment in the health professions as follows:

> The educator must know how the qualitative and quantitative results correlate with the varied stages of learning, as well as with the end goal of graduating a competent fit-for-purpose provider who will not only provide the best care possible, serve the health care needs of communities, but also pass his or her examinations. (p. 187)

I recommend that you rely heavily on faculty colleagues in your program for guidance regarding student assessment as you plan your first few courses. I also recommend that you look closely at the accreditation standards tied to your courses. The verbs in the standards will help you understand how you might go about assessing student competence with a particular standard. For example, if the standard says that the student will "explain" or "describe" something, you can assess student learning through an essay question on an exam. If the standard includes expectations that the student will "apply" or "synthesize," you may need to develop case study assignments or other projects that require these skills. If the standard requires a student to "demonstrate" something, you may need to evaluate the student performing a particular skill via a lab checkout. My program recently completed an extensive program self-study in preparation for reaccreditation. We reviewed how we addressed and assessed each accreditation standard throughout our curriculum. Through this process, my department colleagues and I recognized that, in many cases, we addressed each standard well, but we needed to modify our student assessment strategies to align with student performance expectations outlined in the accreditation standards. We are all much more cognizant now about how we design courses and individual learning activities and assessments, and many times we have said that we wish we had known how to do this when we first became faculty members.

REMEDIATION

No matter how stringent your program's admission guidelines are, you occasionally will have a few students who struggle to maintain the requirements set forth for academic performance and professional behavior. In nearly every cohort I have taught over the past decade, we have had one or two students who struggled for various reasons. Some entered the program with insufficient study skills. Some were great at memorizing but had difficulty with synthesizing information and applying it to case studies and client interactions. Others had inconsistent academic and clinical performance related to health issues and personal stressors. Still others demonstrated great academic performance and clinical skills but did not demonstrate adequate punctuality, attendance, or interpersonal skills.

Your program likely has detailed policies regarding remediation, progression through the program, and requirements for graduation, all of which are required by the accreditation standards for each health professions program (McHugo, 2018). This is another reason to carefully review any handbooks that your program has such as faculty handbooks, student handbooks, or other policy and procedure manuals. If you have a student struggling in one of your courses, you need to address it immediately. I recommend you seek guidance from your department chair or more experienced colleagues before deciding how to proceed, particularly in a cohort-based program. The student may be having issues in other courses as well and may need to set up a remediation plan in order to move forward in the program. Occasionally, students may be dismissed from a health professions program for lack of adequate academic performance, clinical skills, or professional behavior. Despite having a moral obligation to one's own discipline and future potential clients to serve as gatekeepers to the profession, researchers have found a "failure to fail phenomenon" among many health educators and clinical supervisors (Yepes-Rios et al., 2016, p. 1097). Again, if you are not sure what to do with a struggling student, whether in didactic coursework or clinical training, ask for guidance.

PREPARING FOR CLINICALS AND FIELDWORK

In health professions education, everything we do in the classroom leads up to our students working directly with clients across diverse practice settings. Think about the various ways you can prepare students for that transition. Can you introduce them to electronic documentation software that they may encounter at a local hospital or outpatient clinic? Can you have someone from a local school district come to discuss the individualized education plan process for students who receive special education and therapy services? Can you schedule a panel of local clinical educators in your discipline to discuss expectations for clinical skills and professional behaviors? Are there fieldwork resources for students available on your professional association's website? Can you have current students interview students from your program who graduated within the past few years to discuss their clinical experiences? Are your students familiar with the evaluation forms that must be completed by their clinical supervisors? Do they know what to do and who to contact if they are struggling on a particular placement?

DISTANCE LEARNING

If you are teaching a distance education course, you need to familiarize yourself with the instructional tools available through your campus learning management system. There are numerous strategies for designing learning modules, creating lecture capture, facilitating discussion boards and small group collaboration, submitting assignments, and developing online quizzes and exams. Find out if your campus has an educational technology department that provides training for instructors. The learning management system provider for your campus may also have online training available for instructors. Ask other faculty who teach online courses which resources you should explore? You will not have time to learn and implement every tool available to you the first time you teach an online course, but just as if you were teaching in the classroom, you should always be looking for new strategies to incorporate into your teaching.

Course Evaluations

End-of-course evaluations give students the opportunity to provide feedback to instructors anonymously. Many institutions still use the age-old bubble sheets with a section for comments, whereas other institutions have transitioned to online course evaluations. Undoubtedly, you will receive feedback from students disgruntled about their grades or some other aspect of the course. Hopefully, that is mixed with feedback from students who had nothing but positive things to say. If you are really lucky, you will get some constructive feedback that you can use to modify future courses. I have found over the years that I get the most useful feedback when I explain to my students that I value their input, read every comment, and make a few changes each semester. If I am responsible for administering paper evaluations in class, I typically do that at the beginning of a class period rather than the end so students have more time for thoughtful responses and are not worried about getting done as quickly as possible. If your institution administers online course evaluations, find out if you can see how many evaluations have been submitted. A strategy to encourage students to complete the online course evaluations is to offer a few points of extra credit for the entire class if at least 75% of students complete the course evaluations by a particular date. You will not be able to see who has submitted evaluations, but you may be able to see that 25 of 50 evaluations have been submitted. End-of-course evaluation scores and comments are not made available to instructors until after final grades have been posted for the semester.

End-of-course evaluations give you the opportunity to make changes for future courses, but what about making changes that improve the course you are teaching right now? Consider implementing a midsemester course evaluation. This can be something formal via an online or paper survey, or you may consider having students work in small groups to submit written feedback at the end of a particular class period. Another strategy that I learned from my physical therapy colleagues (E. Prost & K. Gibson, personal communication, May 29, 2010) involves having an instructor from another program lead a brief discussion with students focused on two questions: (a) What is going well in the course? and (b) What specific suggestions do you have that would help your learning in this course?

After that session, the faculty member summarizes and discusses the feedback with the course instructor. Then, the course instructor follows up with the students with the following:

- A change that can be made in the current semester
- A change that is not feasible for the current semester but will be taken into consideration for future courses
- An explanation about reasons why you will not consider some of the suggested changes

Regardless of when you obtain feedback from students, you will likely receive some comments that are helpful, some comments that are just complaints about things that you cannot or will not change, and some comments that are just downright mean. I have seen new faculty in tears over hurtful comments from course evaluations.

As a department administrator, I remind students each semester that although we very much value their feedback, there are actual people with feelings who read their comments. I encourage students to provide constructive feedback in a professional manner, just as they would want to be evaluated on their future clinical and field-work rotations. I also remind them to evaluate the course based on the stated course objectives (and accreditation standards, if appropriate) and whether those objectives were met, not so much on whether they liked the course content. Believe me, they will still tell you if they did not like your course, but getting students to understand how faculty use course evaluation data may help you gather more useful feedback.

My department colleagues sometimes get together for happy hour to share selected course comments with one another. It helps to know that others are getting a mix of positive and negative comments. Our department chair also implemented a course reflection process in which we have the opportunity to respond to the evaluations for each course, provide more insight about student responses, and plan changes for future courses if appropriate.

CONCLUSION

This chapter presented only a few ideas that may be useful in your classroom. There are hundreds of other ideas available for use or modification in your particular course. If you have a professional development goal of improving your teaching and increasing student engagement, look for resources specific to these topics. There are entire texts dedicated to instructional strategies and student engagement at the college level. For example, *Student Engagement Techniques: A Handbook for College Faculty* (Barkley, 2010) is an excellent resource that provides 50 specific tips and strategies for fostering motivation, promoting active learning, building community, promoting holistic learning, and ensuring that students are properly challenged. In the same text, Barkley presents 50 student engagement techniques for learning course-related knowledge and skills and developing learner attitudes, values, and self-awareness. Another great resource is *Teaching at Its Best: A Research-Based Resource for College Instructors* (Nilson, 2010). Nilson presents numerous ideas for course design, syllabus development, first day of class activities, preventing and responding to classroom incivility, collaborating with teaching assistants, leading effective discussions, group learning activities, development of student writing skills, and several other topics relevant for college-level teaching.

In addition to resources that address college teaching in general, you should also explore resources within your particular discipline and across the health professions. For example, Plack and Driscoll (2017) presented ideas for understanding ourselves as teachers and our students as learners as well as specific strategies for physical therapy instructors in *Teaching and Learning in Physical Therapy: From Classroom to Clinic, Second Edition*. Sylvia and Barr (2011) take a similar approach in *Pharmacy Education: What Matters in Learning and Teaching*.

You should explore institutional resources available to you. Does your campus have a center for teaching and learning, an educational technology department, or similar entity that provides resources for faculty? If so, go visit the center, talk to the staff, and explore the resources and professional development opportunities. Are there any on-campus conferences related to teaching and learning? If so, make time to attend them, even when you think you simply cannot fit one more thing into your busy schedule.

There are also numerous resources online related to teaching and learning. For example, the Center for Integration of Research, Teaching and Learning (CIRTL; www.cirtl.net) is a collaborative effort between more than 40 research institutions originally funded by the National Science Foundation to improve learning in the science, technology, engineering, and mathematics fields. Faculty in the health professions may find many of the CIRTL resources useful in their own disciplines. In addition to the CIRTL website, many partner institutions have their own CIRTL websites that you can locate through a simple online search.

LEARNING ACTIVITIES

1. Determine whether your campus has a center for teaching and learning. What resources are available to you? Explore online resources from similar centers at other institutions. Begin a list of resources that you would like to explore more in the future.
2. Select a course that you may teach in the future at a particular institution. Locate the course description. What are the expectations of this course? What will students know or be able to do after taking this course? Can you locate a copy of the overall curriculum for this program? How does this course fit into the overall curriculum? Which other courses in the curriculum may be most closely related to this course?
3. Create a syllabus for the course you identified in Learning Activity 2. Does the campus or department have a particular syllabus template that you should use? If you can't locate anything online for this particular institution, try searching for syllabus templates on other institution websites to guide you or follow the list of suggested syllabus content from this chapter.
4. Based on the course syllabus you created, plan learning and assessment activities for one or more class periods. How will you address a specific course objective? How will you assess student learning?
5. Conduct an online search for "tips for large lecture courses." Beyond the few suggestions provided in this chapter, what other ideas did you locate for teaching lecture courses?
6. Conduct an online search for "facilitating student engagement" or "creating community in the college classroom." Beyond the few suggestions provided in this chapter, what other ideas did you locate that you could incorporate into a future course?

7. Search literature in your discipline related to PBL, TBL, and flipped classrooms. Are these strategies that are typically used in educating students in your discipline? What do other educators and scholars have to say about these approaches? Can you think of ways you might incorporate one or more of these strategies into a course you will teach?

8. Identify at least five lab activities for students in your profession. What materials would be required? What would be the optimum number of students for a single faculty member to facilitate in a lab session? What other supports might you need?

9. Explore simulation resources that are relevant for your profession. What is the cost of these resources? What is the benefit of using these resources?

10. Locate a student handbook for a specific program in your discipline, preferably at an institution at which you are interested in teaching. What are the standards for academic performance? Are there remediation policies in place?

11. Imagine you are teaching a course in students' final semester of didactic coursework before they embark on clinicals or fieldwork. Identify at least five learning activities that would help prepare them for the transition from classroom to clinic to entry-level practice.

12. Is distance learning relevant for your profession? If so, explore programs that provide all or some of their curriculum via distance learning. How are those programs structured? What can you find out about course delivery and student expectations?

13. What is the course evaluation process like at your institution? Talk with faculty in your discipline about their experiences with course evaluations. What advice do they have for you regarding the administration of course evaluations and the interpretation of student responses?

REFERENCES

Abdalla, M. E., & Gaffar, A. (2011). *Blueprints in health professions education series—The seven steps of PBL implementation: Tutor manual.* Retrieved from https://www.researchgate.net/publication/235914109_blueprints_in_health_profession_education_series_the_seven_steps_of_pbl_implementation_tutor_manual

Barkley, E. F. (2010). *Student engagement techniques: A handbook for college faculty.* San Francisco, CA: Jossey-Bass.

Berkeley Center for Teaching and Learning. (2019). Considerations for large lecture classes. Retrieved from https://teaching.berkeley.edu/considerations-large-lecture-classes

Brame, C., (2013). Flipping the classroom. Vanderbilt University Center for Teaching. Retrieved from http://cft.vanderbilt.edu/guides-sub-pages/flipping-the-classroom/

Lage, M. J., Platt, G. J., & Treglia, M. (2000). Inverting the classroom: A gateway to creating an inclusive learning environment. *The Journal of Economic Education, 31*(1), 30-43

Lang, J. M. (2012, January 17). Metacognition and student learning. *The Chronicle of Higher Education.* Retrieved from https://www.chronicle.com/article/MetacognitionStudent/130327

Ledlow, S. (2001). Using think-pair-share in the college classroom. University of Notre Dame. Retrieved from https://kaneb.nd.edu/assets/137953/think_pair_share_tips.pdf

McHugo, J. (2018). Learner assessment and remediation. In G. Kayingo & V. M. Hass (Eds.), *The health professions educator: A practical guide for new and established faculty* (pp. 207-219). New York, NY: Springer.

Meckel, M., Cobb, N., Mgobozi, A., Cellissen, E. E., Burrows, K., Riethle, T. J., & Soe, H. Z. (2018). Diverse learner assessment strategies. In G. Kayingo & V. M. Hass (Eds.), *The health professions educator: A practical guide for new and established faculty* (pp. 187-198). New York, NY: Springer.

Nichols, A. A. (2018). Flipping the classroom without tears. In G. Kayingo & V. M. Hass (Eds.), *The health professions educator: A practical guide for new and established faculty* (pp. 79-86). New York, NY: Springer.

Nilson, L. B. (2010). *Teaching at its best: A research-based resource for college instructors.* San Francisco, CA: Jossey-Bass.

Plack, M. M., & Driscoll, M. (2017). *Teaching and learning in physical therapy: From classroom to clinic* (2nd ed.). Thorofare, NJ: SLACK Incorporated.

Sylvia, L. M., & Barr, J. T. (2011). *Pharmacy education: What matters in teaching and learning.* Burlington, MA: Jones and Bartlett Learning.

University of Missouri Faculty Scholars. (2013). Proceedings from UMFS 2012-2013: Integrating Teaching and Scholarship, Lake Ozark, MO.

University of Pittsburgh School of Medicine. (2016). Standardized patient frequently asked questions. Retrieved from http://www.omed.pitt.edu/standardized/faq.php

Walkup, N., Wishner, C., & Gardner, A. (2018). Simulation in clinical education. In G. Kayingo & V. M. Hass (Eds.), *The health professions educator: A practical guide for new and established faculty* (pp. 131-138). New York, NY: Springer Publishing Company.

Wallace, V., & Walker, L. (2018). Team-based learning. In G. Kayingo & V. M. Hass (Eds.), *The health professions educator: A practical guide for new and established faculty* (pp. 67-78). New York, NY: Springer.

Yepes-Rios, M., Dudek, N., Duboyce, R., Curtis, J., Allard, R. J., & Varpio, L. (2016). The failure to fail underperforming trainees in health professions education: A BEME systematic review: BEME Guide No. 42. *Medical Teacher, 38*(11), 1092-1099. doi:10.1080/0142159X.2016.1215414

12

Facilitating Professional Behavior Development in Students

Before we begin thinking about professional behavior, let's step back and ask ourselves, "What is a profession?" This topic has been discussed in academia for more than a century. In 1910, Abraham Flexner, known for his work in reforming medical education, identified the following six characteristics of a profession (Flexner, 1910):

1. Professions involve intellectual activity and individual responsibility.
2. Professional knowledge is based on scientific learning.
3. Professional activity involves practical application, not just theorizing.
4. Professions have their own language and techniques that can be taught.
5. Professions tend to have internal organizations (e.g., professional associations).
6. Professions are motivated by altruism, working for the good of society.

In historical context, the *Flexner Report* is viewed controversially, with some hailing his work as the greatest contribution to U.S. medical education (Seyal, 2013), whereas others describe him as sexist and racist (Hiatt, 1999). Regardless of the controversy surrounding his work, Flexner was instrumental in establishing high standards for the educational preparation of physicians. As other health professions developed, they followed similar practices in establishing educational requirements to prepare individuals for professional practice (Thibault, 2013).

In contemporary health professions education, didactic and clinical education is guided by standards of practice, educational accreditation standards, and codes of ethics established by each profession. Undoubtedly, the students in your health professions programs will have some desire to help others, or they would not be pursuing a degree in the health professions.

Gateley, C. A. *Clinical Practice to Academia: A Guide for New and Aspiring Health Professions Faculty* (pp. 175-190). © 2021 Taylor & Francis Group.

Each profession is characterized by having practitioners expressing a common core of professional attributes that are characteristic of professionals. Other attributes tend to be innate in those who tend to seek entry into specific programs. Still other attributes are desired and may be enhanced through training. (Missouri State University, 2017, para. 24)

In my experience, it is the final sentence of the previous quote that leads to frustration among both new and seasoned faculty because their expectations of professional behavior clash drastically with the behaviors demonstrated by many students in their classes. This chapter explores many of those issues and offers a few suggestions as you transition into a faculty role.

Transitioning From Prerequisite Coursework to a Professional Program

When I began my occupational therapy educational program in 1992, I never would have considered showing up late for class, skipping class, turning in assignments late, or arguing with a professor about a grade. Admittedly, I have always been a rule follower, but those behaviors were rarely demonstrated by any of the students in my cohort. When I began my full-time faculty position at my alma mater in 2009, I was astonished at the change in students' attitudes and behaviors. Students often missed class for various reasons ranging from illness to vacation to participation in recreational soccer games to planned hangovers. I actually received the following email from a student: "Hey Crystal, Tuesday is my 21st birthday so I'm probably not gonna feel like coming to class Wednesday morning." Students argued with me for every point deducted on assignments and exams. The following is an actual statement from a student who received a 90% on her very first assignment in a clinical documentation course: "I even had my Mom review this assignment. She works in health care, and she said it was perfect. Maybe if YOU provided a better grading rubric, we'd understand what you want from us." For the record, I kept this student after class and explained to her that if she were my student out on a clinical rotation, I would have dismissed her from the rotation on the spot for her lack of professionalism and insubordinate behavior. Two years later at graduation, she told me that conversation was one of the most memorable and important events in her college experience and professional development.

I began conducting research among my own students to better understand why they thought and behaved the way they did. One student wrote the following:

I got through my prerequisite coursework with going to class occasionally and minimal studying, and I still got mostly As and Bs. I got into this [occupational therapy] program, and you expected me to be here every day, on time. And you expected me to actually do the readings you assigned. That was a really hard transition for me.

I was stunned. I viewed showing up to class on time and prepared as an unspoken expectation for a professional program. What I have learned over the past 10 years is that faculty and administrators have to be very explicit in communicating expectations for professional behavior in individual classes and across professional programs. Each year I see more students in my program struggle with professional behaviors than academic or clinical performance.

TIME MANAGEMENT AND CLASS PREPARATION

Many students enter health professions education programs without the essential study skills necessary for success in a rigorous curriculum. Across higher education, it is common practice that for every 1 credit hour of coursework, faculty expect students to spend 2 to 3 hours outside of class reading, studying, completing assignments, or otherwise preparing for class (Bennett, 2000; University of Michigan–Flint, 2018). For students enrolled in 15 credit hours, that translates into 30 to 45 hours of preparation outside of class. However, the National Survey for Student Engagement suggests that today's full-time college students spend only about 17 hours per week preparing for classes (Pierre, 2014).

In my own program, I see a similar pattern each year. Individual faculty discuss these expectations with students in each course at the beginning of the semester. We include discussion about successful study habits during an orientation program as students enter our program. I even have had panels of former students who took each class come talk to current students about what to expect and how to be successful. Then, about 3 to 4 weeks into each semester, about the time when students have their first round of exams, mild to moderate panic sets in as many students become overwhelmed with the amount of reading, studying, and homework that they have across our professional curriculum. Although I do think it helpful to try to prepare students with the methods I described earlier, most students admit that they just did not get it until they were partway through the semester and realized they had to make some adjustments to their schedules.

During a recent semester, when I began to get the "What suggestions do you have for being successful in your class?" question from frustrated students, I asked their peers for feedback rather than simply repeating the advice I had already given at the beginning of the semester. I looked at the overall course grades, sent out an email to all students who were performing at the A level in my courses, asked for their advice for classmates, and compiled their responses. I posted that information for all students on Canvas (our campus learning management system), and we held a class discussion for about 30 minutes. Many students reported that they had to drop some extracurricular activities or reduce their work commitment. Successful students also reported that they scheduled time for studying each day rather than trying to cram immediately before an exam. Students also offered a variety of other suggestions about how they studied for each exam. Several students stopped me after class or emailed me to thank me for taking time to address their concerns. Additionally, the students who were asked to provide advice were pleased that their performance had been recognized and that their input was valued.

Social Media

Most students in your classrooms cannot remember a time without Facebook, Twitter, Instagram, Snapchat, and all the other social media platforms available today. They have grown up posting pictures and videos of themselves and their events on a daily basis. Many of them need to be reminded to clean up their social media presence when they enter a professional program because they are no longer just representing themselves. They now represent your program and your profession. One of my favorite activities to make new students in our program more aware of how they present themselves online is to randomly divide the class into small groups and tell them that they have been placed in those groups based on some commonalities that I was able to identify after searching their online presence. This activity serves two purposes. First, many students are stunned that their professor would "stalk" them online and worried about what I may have seen. Second, most groups manage to find something that they all have in common, even if they have never met before. After the activity, I tell them that I do not have the time nor interest in stalking their online profiles, but any of their future clinical supervisors or potential employers might do exactly that.

Many institutions and health professions educational programs now have social media policies in place to guide students, staff, and faculty in the appropriate use of social media. You need to be familiar with the policies at your institution, and you need to educate students regarding those policies. One very important issue to discuss with them is maintaining client privacy. The Health Insurance Portability and Accountability Act of 1996 (HIPAA) provides standards for maintaining privacy of health information across all health professions and settings (U.S. Department of Health & Human Services, 2013). Most students have heard of HIPAA, but they may not understand how easily they can violate HIPAA guidelines with a simple social media post. There are numerous resources online that you can incorporate into your coursework to help students better understand this concept.

Academic Dishonesty

Academic dishonesty has risen drastically over the past several decades. Researchers report that approximately 75% to 90% of students have cheated at some point during their time in college (American College Personnel Association [ACPA], 2015; Best College Reviews, 2018; Dimon, 2018; Jaffe, 2018). Most of those students have been cheating occasionally or often since middle or high school.

> While academic dishonesty can take many forms—from using a "cheat sheet" on an exam to plagiarizing an entire research paper—cheating is detrimental not only to the student who engages in the behavior, but to the field of higher education as a whole. Higher education institutions assist in students' development in various areas, including ethical development and understanding of rigorous academic and research standards . . . student cheating is at odds with this mission. (ACPA, 2015, para. 1)

Why do students cheat? The reasons are endless, but following is a list of some of the most common reasons identified by recent research into this academic dishonesty (ACPA, 2015; Best College Reviews, 2018; Jaffe, 2018; Simkin & McLeod, 2010):

- Lack of understanding about what constitutes cheating
- Desire to succeed
- Little or no desire to put in the required effort
- Time demands
- Low risk of getting caught
- Gains outweigh potential penalties
- Low perceived value of class or assignment
- Pressure from parents or self-imposed pressure for high performance
- Peer pressure, particularly among high-achieving students being asked to help other students cheat
- Emphasis on grades rather than learning
- Diversity of moral codes, with some students seeing nothing wrong with cheating
- Easily accessible opportunities, such as online paper mills
- Faculty who are reluctant to enforce consequences

The ways in which students cheat are as diverse as their reasons for doing it (ACPA, 2015; Best College Reviews, 2018; Jaffe, 2018; Simkin & McLeod, 2010). When I was an undergraduate back in the 1990s, opportunities for cheating were limited to just a few options like sneaking notes into an exam, plagiarizing material without properly citing or paraphrasing, accessing "test banks" in sororities and fraternities, and paying someone else to complete the work. With technological advances, students now have numerous other ways to cheat in college. They can order papers online for nearly any subject. They can pay a monthly subscription for unlimited answers to math and science problems. They can easily share answers with each other through email and cell phones. Several years ago, a colleague at my institution found a group of students sitting together completing what was intended to be an individual online quiz. Although the questions were presented in random order for each student, together they were able to ensure that each of them got all or most of the answers correct. Eliminating technology during in-class exams can reduce cheating, but students are very creative. Even though you may tell them to put away their cell phones and laptops, monitoring the activity of a large classroom can be challenging for an instructor when students can easily hide a cell phone in their lap or leave it partially concealed in a backpack.

The advent of smartwatches and other wireless technology also poses new opportunities for cheating. Recently, I had students who mentioned on end-of-course evaluations that there were students in the class who were concealing wireless earbuds under their long hair and listening to recorded notes during in-class exams and assignments. Other students find new ways to use old methods of cheating by having notes written in the bill of their hats, concealed on water bottle labels, or tucked into their underwear. A few years ago, we had a student in our program who needed to "use the restroom" during nearly every exam in every course. Our faculty implemented a no bathroom policy during exams and encouraged students to go take care of business immediately before beginning the exam so there would be no reason to leave class during the exam.

ATTENDANCE AND PUNCTUALITY

As an undergraduate in the 1990s, skipping class or showing up late never crossed my mind. There were certainly students in my larger lecture classes during prerequisite coursework who skipped classes on a regular basis, but once I entered my professional program, students rarely missed a class. Today, skipping class is commonplace.

> Studies show that class attendance is the number one predictor of grades in a college course, outranking time spent studying, studying skills, high school grades or standardized tests. Despite this clear connection, even the most optimistic academic studies find that nearly one in five U.S. college students are skipping on any given day—with absentee rates reaching up to 70 percent for some large classes at major state universities. (College Planning & Management, 2015, para. 9)

According to a recent study, students' top reasons for skipping class are hanging out with friends, fatigue, participating in a recreational event, studying for another class, and weather (College Planning & Management, 2015). Having taught at the college level for over a decade, I can assure you that those are not the same reasons students provide to their instructors. In large lecture undergraduate courses, where students may or may not communicate with the instructor about why they missed a class, students most frequently told me they were sick or had some sort of personal emergency. Another common excuse is "My cell phone alarm didn't go off." In my smaller professional program courses, students often tell me in advance that they are going to miss class for a family event or travel plans. Keep in mind that most of your students experienced K–12 education where a note or phone call from a parent was all that was needed for an "excused absence" and that it was common for parents to pull students out of school for up to a week or more for vacation in the middle of the school year (Ortiz, 2017).

I continuously have modified my attendance policies in my professional-level courses over the years to help students develop the professional behaviors required for entry-level practice in the health professions. Your department may have an attendance policy that is used across all courses, or you may have sole discretion in setting attendance policies for your courses. When I first started teaching full time, I inherited a course and syllabus from another professor who gave "attendance points" for each class period. I later determined that those attendance points cushioned students' overall course grades so much that there was little distinction between average, good, and excellent performance.

The following semester, I no longer gave attendance points. I viewed attending class as a basic requirement, but I also understood that students do occasionally have legitimate reasons for missing a class, such as an illness or personal emergency. I stated the following in my syllabi: "You are adults, and I assume that whatever reason you have for missing class was important to you." I allowed students one absence without consequence. I quickly learned that students will take what you give them. By the end of the semester, nearly every student had been sick or had a broken-down vehicle at least one time. One student even emailed me and said, "Hey, I'm going to take my free absence tomorrow because the weather is great and I just want to spend the day outside. Are you going over anything important in class?" Free absence? Isn't everything I cover important? I originally thought I had improved my attendance policy while allowing some grace for unexpected events, but all I had done was given students a sense of entitlement to a personal day to use as they wished.

My next change was to implement a consequence for missing a class. On the first absence, regardless of the reason, students had the choice to lose 10 points (about 2% of the course grade) or complete a makeup assignment, typically an article review over the topic covered in the missed class. Any subsequent absences, regardless of the reason, resulted in an automatic 10-point deduction without opportunity to make up those points. During the first few years with this policy, I saw nearly a 90% drop in absenteeism compared to my previous policies. Rather than most students missing at least one class period, only a few students ever missed class. Then, over the next several years, I again saw changes in the pattern of students' behavior. More and more students were choosing to do the makeup assignment so they could have their personal day. This created more work for me to develop and grade extra assignments beyond those outlined in the course syllabus.

My current attendance policy is that there is a point deduction for every absence without opportunity to make up the points. The point deduction varies depending on how many total points are in the course. I typically have the first absence worth only about 2% of the overall course grade, which is not enough to significantly affect the grade of a student who is otherwise performing well in the course and has a legitimate illness or personal situation. Subsequent absences are 5% of the overall course grade, which can quickly add up to trouble for students in a graduate or professional program where academic standards often require that they maintain at least a B in all coursework. With this policy, my absentee rate is back down again with only a couple absences per semester across each course. I also now have a similar tardiness policy because the number of students who do not make it to class on time has been an increasing issue in recent years.

The policies I described previously were in graduate and professional coursework where my class sizes ranged from 30 to 45 students, and I knew the students well because I had them in multiple courses over 2 to 3 years. Large undergraduate courses are very different. In a lecture hall with hundreds of students, instructors have much more difficulty tracking attendance and managing the dozens of emails about absences over the course of the semester. Some faculty use student response systems, such as iClickers (Macmillan Learning), to take attendance or give in-class quizzes. Others may require students to "swipe in" with their student identification card to verify attendance. Still others do not have a set policy and instead assume that grades will sort themselves out when students who miss many classes perform poorly on exams.

When you begin a new faculty position, be sure to find out if there are departmental guidelines that you need to follow regarding attendance policies. If you have autonomy in establishing your own policies, ask for help! Talk to other faculty within your department or school to see which policies work well for them. Ask if you can borrow their attendance policy wording for your own syllabi. Regardless of which policy you implement, you likely will make changes over the course of time. Additionally, for every policy in place, there are usually a few rare exceptions. For example, I do not penalize students for missing class to attend a funeral; however, I do not tell the class this information up front because unfortunately there are students who falsely will claim to have lost a loved one if they know in advance they will not be penalized for the absence. I also have had students who had a parent with cancer, who lacked day care options when their child was ill, or who were dealing with some serious physical or mental health concerns, and I allowed a bit more flexibility with my attendance policy in those situations. Students also should not be penalized for jury duty, military service, or observance of religious holidays.

Making exceptions to your attendance policies beyond the circumstances described earlier can be a slippery slope. If a student is in a wedding and has to miss class to travel out of town and arrive on time for the rehearsal, that seems like a legitimate excuse, right? But what about the student whose parents scheduled a family vacation in the middle of the semester and already purchased a plane ticket? Beyond obvious personal emergencies, I try to avoid putting myself in the position of having to decide which reasons are worthy of missing my class by adhering strictly to the attendance policies presented at the beginning of the semester. Students will talk among themselves and before you know it, students are complaining to a department chair or dean about perceived inequity in treatment. When in doubt, ask for guidance from experienced colleagues and your department chair. If a student does question you directly about how you handled another student's absence, you can simply say that the Family Educational Rights and Privacy Act prevents you from discussing another student's situation.

If you have student athletes in any of your courses, you may need to make additional exceptions to your attendance policies. Although I am certain practices vary somewhat across institutions, my experience with student athletes has always been very positive. Student athletes or a representative from the athletic department should communicate with you early in the semester about upcoming absences and to make arrangements about making up missed work or exams. Keep in mind that student athletes are often receiving a scholarship in return for their athletic participation for the institution. They also typically have advisors and academic supports in place to keep them on track with their academic requirements so that they remain eligible to compete in their sport. If you find that a student athlete's absences are affecting academic or clinical performance in your program, address those issues immediately with the student, the athletic support staff, and/or your department chair.

You may also have students enrolled in your course who have flexible attendance accommodations through the office of disability services. This topic was also discussed in Chapter 9. You will need to work directly with the student and his or her disability advisor to determine what flexible attendance means for your particular course.

COMMUNICATION SKILLS

Students accepted into health professions programs bring with them vastly different levels of interpersonal and professional communication skills. They likely have had some form of speech or communications course, and they impressed the admissions committee with their written application and interview, but most students still need guidance about how to communicate with others in a way that matches your expectations of an entry-level health care professional. Do not make the mistake of assuming that your students know what appropriate communication skills are in the classroom or clinical setting. If good communication skills were innate, there would not be entire textbooks devoted to the development of communication skills in health professions students. McCorry and Mason (2011) reviewed the communication process, verbal and nonverbal communication with clients and other health care professionals, client interviewing techniques, adapting communication skills to the client's ability to understand for improved health literacy, cultural sensitivity in health care communication, and electronic communications skills. It is beyond the scope of this book to go in depth into all of these topics, but I would like to focus on a few key points that you may need to emphasize with students.

Students may not know how to properly format an email to you as an instructor. Corrigan and McNabb (2016) explained the following:

> In the age of social media, many students approach emailing similar to texting and other forms of digital communication, where the crucial conventions are brevity and informality. But most college teachers consider emails closer to letters than to text messages. (para. 3)

They recommend the following strategies to help students' email communications be perceived as more professional by their instructors, and I recommend including this information for students in your syllabus or on your course management site (e.g., Canvas, Blackboard) to reduce awkward encounters later on:

- Use a clear subject line such as "Research Paper #1" rather than "Heeeelllpp!" or leaving the subject line blank.
- Use a salutation and appropriate title. Do not begin with "Hey, Crystal!" Instead, use "Good Morning, Professor Gateley" or "Good Afternoon, Dr. Gateley." I have seen significant differences in expectations about what instructors wish to be called. Some professors expect to be called "Dr." if they have earned any form of doctorate degree. Some departments require students to address all instructors as "Professor" because faculty may have different academic degrees. In some graduate and professional programs, students and faculty may interact on a first name basis. If there is this much discrepancy across institutions and between departments, it is no wonder that students often make mistakes. Make it easy for your students. Tell them how you wish to be addressed in person and in email communication.

- Use standard punctuation, spelling, capitalization, and grammar. Do not use common texting abbreviations.
- Do your part in solving your problem. Do not ask the instructor for information that you can readily locate in the syllabus or on the course management system.
- Be careful not to sound entitled. "If you appear to demand help, shrug off absences or assume late work will be accepted without penalty because you have a good reason, your professors may see you as irresponsible or presumptuous" (Corrigan & McNabb, 2016, para. 10).
- Add a touch of humanity by commenting on something covered in class or perhaps an outside connection you have made to the course material.

Students also may not recognize boundaries in how and what they say to a professor or classmate. There is a big difference between respectfully debating a difference of opinion and being offensive or confrontational about something you disagree with, whether it be the opinion of the professor or a classmate or the grade received on an assignment. NIU Faculty Development (2010) recommended establishing expectations for mutually respectful communications in the syllabus and by discussing expectations on the first day of class. Students expect you to set rules for classroom decorum. "The more proactive you are in establishing your expectations, the less likely it is that you will have to respond to uncivil behaviors" (NIU Faculty Development, 2010). Additionally, faculty should model respectful communication and step in when things go awry in the classroom.

Any situations that disrupt the learning environment or threaten the safety of the student or instructor must be dealt with immediately. If the student's inappropriate communication or behavior is brief and you can move on with the class without further disruption, speak to the student in private after class. NIU Faculty Development (2010) recommends first asking if the student is okay to show concern for the student's well-being and be prepared to refer the student to the student health center or student counseling center if needed. If there is no immediate health problem, you should include the following four elements in your conversation with the student (NIU Faculty Development, 2010):

1. Begin by specifically identifying the problematic behavior. Avoid phrases like "what do you think you're doing?" If possible, use the student's name.
2. Briefly explain why the behavior is problematic. This may be because it distracts others or because it is in violation of the rules for classroom deportment you have established.
3. Request that the behavior cease.
4. Identify what actions you will be compelled to take if the behavior doesn't cease (NIU Faculty Development, 2010).

Beyond classroom incivility, students may demonstrate inappropriate communication skills in email communications with professors or online discussion forums with classmates. These students often have limited self-awareness about how their interactions are perceived by others. Unless you want to deal with frustrated clinical instructors when your students go out for their clinical rotations and other experiential learning, you need to have difficult conversations with students when these situations arise so they better understand how their communication skills can affect their overall professionalism and success as a student and future health care professional.

DRESS CODE

Think about different jobs you have had throughout your life. Were there different expectations about what you were expected to wear to each of those jobs? How did you find out what the rules were? Were there ever examples of individuals who pushed the limits of acceptable attire? What were the consequences?

Although appropriate attire for a health care setting may seem like common sense to someone reading this book, do not assume that your students understand the rules. Most health professions programs have a specific dress code policy or student handbook that delineates expectations for students in the classroom and clinical environment. For example, the University of Arizona College of Medicine (2016) explained the following:

> Students have freedom of choice in how they dress. However, when students are functioning as medical professionals, with either clinical patients or simulated patients, or in-classroom in nonclinical settings, dress must be appropriate and professional. A professional image increases credibility and safety while fostering patient trust, respect and confidence. Non-adherence to the dress code can have negative effects on patient care and could diminish the reputation of the medical school, as well affiliated hospitals and clinics. (p. 1)

Simply explaining the purpose behind professional dress code is not enough. Health professions programs typically provide specific examples of what is and is not acceptable in the classroom or clinical setting. For example, students may need to be told that shorts, leggings, athletic pants, and non-collared shirts are not appropriate for clinical settings.

Any program in which you accept a faculty position likely will already have a dress code policy in place. As a new faculty member, you should familiarize yourself with the policy and be prepared to coach students when they do not follow the established guidelines. You should also incorporate expectations for professional dress into occasional classroom assignments, like presentations and mock interviews, so students get the opportunity to practice their professional behavior skills and receive faculty feedback rather than making errors in a clinical setting that could impact how they are viewed by clients and clinical supervisors.

RECOGNIZING BIAS

The importance of respecting individual differences is widely recognized as a basic tenet of being a health care professional. You might think that individuals who enter the health professions are more open minded than the general population about differences they may encounter in their clients. However, a recent systematic review of literature on this topic revealed that "healthcare professionals exhibit the same levels of implicit bias as the wider population" (Fitzgerald & Hurst, 2017, p. 19). Knowing that such biases contribute to health care disparities, part of our job as health professions faculty is to help students recognize their own implicit biases about race, ethnicity, socioeconomic status, gender identity, sexual orientation, weight, disability, mental illness, addiction, social circumstance, and a myriad of other factors that may affect how they view and treat their future clients. Sukhera and Watling (2018) proposed "a six-point actionable framework for integrating implicit bias recognition and management into health professions education that draws on the work of previous researchers and includes practical tools to guide curriculum developers" (p. 35). The key points of the framework include the following:

- Creating a safe and nonthreatening learning context: Teaching and learning about implicit bias is challenging. Students need an approachable instructor who addresses the discomfort that accompanies difficult conversations and reflections about bias and privilege. "A key distinction between traditional education about diversity or cultural competence and implicit-bias-informed curricula is a proactive shift away from guilt and toward responsibility" (Sukhera & Watling, 2018, p. 36). Students need sufficient time to grapple with complex issues, and they need to know that their confidentiality regarding classroom discussions and reflection papers or other assignments will be respected by instructors and classmates.

- Increasing knowledge about the science of implicit bias: Students need to understand the psychological and neurobiological components of bias in order to recognize that eliminating bias is impossible.

- Emphasizing how implicit bias influences behaviors and patient outcomes: Providing students with evidence on how sociocultural forces can influence health disparities, clinical decision making, and patient safety may motivate them to recognize and address their own biases. You may be able to find evidence on these topics for your specific discipline, or you may need to rely on evidence from other health professions.

- Increasing self-awareness of existing implicit biases: There are numerous resources available online for activities that help students recognize and reflect on their own identity, privilege, and implicit biases. For example, Sukhera and Watling (2018) recommended using the Implicit Association Test available on the Harvard University website as a starting point for reflective discussions. You may also have campus resources that can assist you in developing activities to address these issues.

- Improving conscious efforts to overcome implicit bias: When students recognize that they have biases, they want to know how to address them. One strategy is helping students understand metacognition, or how to think about their thinking. Additionally, learning mindfulness techniques and implementing strategies for self-monitoring over time can help students recognize progress they have made over time in addressing their implicit biases.

- Enhancing awareness of how implicit bias influences others: Beyond self-awareness of their own biases, students need to understand how others are impacted by bias. Giving students opportunities to understand the perspectives of others can help them develop empathy for individuals from different backgrounds and change the way they perceive and interact with them. Examples of strategies for enhancing student understanding include role play, social contact with individuals from marginalized groups, and stories and videos about marginalized groups.

Sukhera and Watling (2018) cautioned that implicit bias cannot be sufficiently addressed in a single class session or even in a single course. Rather, faculty need to decide how bias-informed educational approaches should be integrated throughout a curriculum and how student outcomes and program outcomes will be assessed.

Transitioning From a Professional Program to Clinicals and Entry-Level Practice

Many health professions education programs have clinical, fieldwork, or practicum experiences integrated throughout their curricula. Examples include spending a few hours, days, weeks, or even months at a hospital, clinic, or other setting relevant to the discipline. These experiences give students the opportunity to put together all the aspects of professional behavior discussed in this chapter. Despite all the emphasis you and your academic colleagues may have placed on the importance of professional behaviors, students are likely to be more concerned about whether they can demonstrate the necessary clinical skills on their rotations than about any challenges they may encounter about professional behavior. In my experience, students tend to listen more to peers, recent graduates, clinical supervisors, and potential employers than their professors when it comes to issues related to professionalism. Ask students to provide examples, perhaps anonymously, of issues related to professional behavior that they witnessed or personally encountered during clinical experiences, and use these examples as talking points for class discussion. Bring in a panel of current clinical instructors, fieldwork educators, or whatever the appropriate term is for your profession, and ask them to talk with students about the mistakes they have seen students make in the past related to professional behavior. Bring in a panel of local managers from settings relevant to your profession and ask them to discuss facility policies related to attendance, tardiness, dress code, and other aspects related to professional behavior.

Learning Activities

1. Locate the educational accreditation standards for your profession. What mention do you find regarding professional behavior?
2. Locate the standards of practice and/or code of ethics for your profession. (Note that some professions may use different terminology, but these keywords should yield a similar document). What are the expectations of professionals in your discipline?

3. Conduct a search using the terms "professional behavior" and your discipline. Read one or more of the sources and discuss with classmates the issues that are prominent in your profession.

4. Conduct a search using the terms "professional behavior" and "college students." Read one or more of the sources and discuss with classmates the issues that are prominent in higher education.

5. Make a list of unprofessional behaviors that you have witnessed in your time as a college student or perhaps are even guilty of yourself.

6. On average, how many hours per week do you (or did you) spend studying and preparing for each class?

7. If you are currently enrolled in a course, discuss with classmates strategies you have found most helpful for academic success throughout your higher education journey.

8. Conduct a search for social media policies or guidelines at your institution or one at which you are interested in working and compare what you found with your classmates.

9. Conduct a search using the keywords "social media" and "HIPAA." What examples of HIPAA violations did you learn about?

10. Conduct a search for policies related to academic dishonesty at your institution or one where you may pursue a faculty position. What constitutes academic dishonesty? What are your responsibilities as a faculty member in dealing with suspected academic dishonesty? What consequences might a student face for engaging in academic dishonesty?

11. Conduct a search with key phrases such as "pay someone to write my paper" or "pay someone to take my class." What did you find?

12. Discuss with classmates times that you or someone you know has cheated in college. Why did you do it? How did you do it? What would you do if you caught one of your students cheating?

13. Conduct a search for "sample syllabus attendance policies." Discuss with your classmates which policies you believe would be most effective in encouraging students to attend class regularly.

14. Conduct a search for "student dress code" within your discipline. Review some of the policies that you found. What commonalities can you identify?

15. Conduct a search for "activities to help students identify bias" or "activities to help students identify privilege." Did you find any activities that you believe would be relevant for students in your health profession?

16. Select a college or university that you may potentially teach at in the future. Conduct an online search about campus resources that may be available to address issues related to bias. Try searching for "office of diversity and inclusion" or using similar key terms. What resources did you find that could be incorporated into learning activities for students in your discipline?

17. Contact someone who currently practices in your profession. Ask about policies related to attendance, dress code, and other aspects of professionalism. Ask "What do you wish students or new practitioners would do differently when they come to your setting?" Discuss your results with classmates. Are there any common themes?

REFERENCES

American College Personnel Association. (2015, June 1.) The cheating epidemic: Reducing academically dishonest behaviors among college students. Retrieved from http://www.myacpa.org/article/cheating-epidemic-reducing-academically-dishonest-behaviors-amongst-college-students

Bennett, J. (2000). Hints on how to succeed in college classes. UC Sand Diego. Retrieved from https://caps.ucsd.edu/Downloads/tx_forms/koch/college_success/college_success.pdf

Best College Reviews. (2018). Cheating in college: The numbers and research. Retrieved from https://www.bestcollegereviews.org/cheating/

College Planning & Management. (2015, August 6). College students reveal why they skip class in 140 characters or less. Spaces4Learning. Retrieved from https://webcpm.com/articles/2015/08/06/why-college-students-skip-class.aspx

Corrigan, P., & McNabb, C. H. (2016, October 20). Re: your recent email to your professor. Chatfield College. Retrieved from https://chatfield.edu/re-recent-email-professor/

Dimon, M. (2018). 90% of college students have cheated. University Magazine. Retrieved from https://universitymagazine.ca/90-percent-college-students-cheated/

Fitzgerald, C., & Hurst, S. (2017). Implicit bias in health care professionals: A systematic review. *BMC Medical Ethics, 18,* 19. doi: 10.1186/s12910-017-0179-8

Flexner, A. (1910). *Medical education in the United States and Canada: A report to the Carnegie Foundation for the Advancement of Teaching.* Carnegie Foundation for the Advancement of Teaching. Retrieved from http://archive.carnegiefoundation.org/pdfs/elibrary/Carnegie_Flexner_Report.pdf

Hiatt, M. D. (1999). Around the continent in 180 days: The controversial journey of Abraham Flexner. *Pharos, 62*(1), 18-24.

Jaffe, D. (2018). Academic cheating fact sheet. Stanford University. Retrieved from https://web.stanford.edu/class/engr110/cheating.html

McCorry, L. K., & Mason, J. (2011). *Communication skills for the healthcare professional.* Philadelphia, PA: Lippincott Williams & Wilkins.

Missouri State University. (2017). *Professionalism in the health sciences: Definitions, rights, and responsibilities.* Retrieved from https://www.missouristate.edu/bms/CMB/Professionalism.htm

NIU Faculty Development. (2010, October 6). *Promoting and Maintaining Classroom Civility* [Video]. YouTube. https://www.youtube.com/watch?v=nSyFyKK0Iy8&t=774s

Ortiz, V. (2017, April 11). Schools crack down on absences for vacations. *Chicago Tribune.* Retrieved from https://www.chicagotribune.com/news/ct-school-absences-vacations-met-20170410-story.html

Pierre, K. (2014, August 18). How much do you study? Apparently 17 hours per week is the norm. *USA Today.* Retrieved from https://www.usatoday.com/story/college/2014/08/18/how-much-do-you-study-apparently-17-hours-a-week-is-the-norm/37395213/

Seyal, M. S. (2013). Abraham Flexner: His life and legacy. *Hektoen International: A Journal of Medical Humanities, 5*(3), 1.

Simkin, M. G., & McLeod, A. (2010). Why do college students cheat? *Journal of Business Ethics, 94*(3), 441-453. doi:10.1007/s10551-009-0275-x

Sukhera, J., & Watling, C. (2018). A framework for integrating implicit bias into health professions education. *Academic Medicine, 93*(1), 35-40. doi:10.1097/ACM.0000000000001819.

Thibault, G. E. (2013). Reforming health professions education will require culture change and closer ties between classroom and practice. *Health Affairs, 32*(11), 1. doi:10.1377/hlthaff.2013.0827

University of Arizona College of Medicine. (2016). *Medical student dress code policy.* Retrieved from https://medicine.arizona.edu/sites/default/files/dress_code_policy_rev_11.29.16.pdf

University of Michigan–Flint. (2018). *Surviving college.* Retrieved from https://www.umflint.edu/advising/surviving_college

U.S. Department of Health & Human Services. (2013). *Summary of the HIPAA Privacy Rule.* Retrieved from https://www.hhs.gov/hipaa/for-professionals/privacy/laws-regulations/index.html

13

Professional Development for Health Professions Faculty

Most health professions require practitioners to accrue a particular number of continuing education hours every year or two to maintain national certification and/ or state licensure. Health professionals typically seek out additional training related to the specific setting in which they work. For example, a respiratory therapist working in a hospital may attend a weekend course about recent advances in respiratory care for clients with chronic obstructive pulmonary disorder. A speech-language pathologist working in a school setting may attend a conference about addressing articulation disorders in young children. An occupational therapist working at an outpatient orthopedic clinic may pursue advanced certification as a hand therapist. You will need to maintain the same national certification and state licensure in academia as you do in clinical practice, but your learning needs likely will have changed somewhat. Although it is still important to stay up to date with current practices in your profession, you will also benefit from professional development specifically related to your role as a faculty member. Check your profession's requirements carefully to determine which type of professional development events will count toward maintaining your credentials and licensure. There are numerous opportunities for professional development related to teaching and other academic responsibilities.

Gateley, C. A. *Clinical Practice to Academia: A Guide for New and Aspiring Health Professions Faculty* (pp. 191-197). © 2021 Taylor & Francis Group.

SEEKING OUT PROFESSIONAL DEVELOPMENT OPPORTUNITIES

Professional development opportunities that will be beneficial to you in your new role as a faculty member will not come neatly packaged for you in a list to be checked off. You will encounter some of them by chance, and some of them you will find out about through intentional searching. The following are a few of the ways you may hear about potential professional opportunities:

- Read your email: You likely will receive daily or weekly emails that are distributed campus wide to all faculty. A lot of the information contained in such emails will not be relevant to you, but it is worth your time to skim these emails for campus programs and workshops related to teaching and research. Over the years, I have learned of several campus workshops in this manner, with topics ranging from the use of technology in the classroom to requirements for submitting research proposals to the institutional review board. When I see a program of interest to me, I put it on my electronic calendar, even if I am not positive that I will be able to attend when the date arrives. Other opportunities require more planning and commitment. For example, several years ago I learned via email about a faculty development program called University of Missouri Faculty Scholars, which was "designed to support the efforts of the university to acclimate and retain new faculty members" (University of Missouri System, 2016). This year-long program involved campus-specific activities and three system-wide retreats, and participation involved a competitive application process as well as a letter of support from my department chair.

- Ask others for advice: Talk to your department chair and other faculty within your department and school. Ask if they have recommendations about particular programs or activities that will help you develop your skills as a new college educator. They may be aware of programs that occur only once or twice per year that you otherwise would not learn about for months if you rely solely on email notifications. For example, through informal conversations during my first year, I learned about the Wakonse Conference on College Teaching, a 4-day retreat sponsored by my university that brings together faculty and academic professionals from dozens of institutions to share insights, experiences, and practical strategies for enhancing teaching and learning (University of Missouri Career Center, 2019).

- Do some online exploration: Explore your school and campus websites to search for resources related to teaching and research. Your campus may have resources related to teaching or educational technology that will help you in your new role. If resources on your campus are limited, search the websites of other colleges and universities that may provide free online resources to faculty. You should also check the websites of professional organizations relevant to your discipline to see if there are resources for college educators that may be of benefit to you.

CENTERS FOR TEACHING AND LEARNING

Find out if your campus has a center for teaching and learning, and, if so, thoroughly explore its resources and programs. If your campus does not have such a center, do a Google search for "university center for teaching," and you will get hundreds of results. Explore the websites of centers on your campus and other centers to locate useful information for your role as a new college educator. For example, the website for Vanderbilt University's Center for Teaching has links to numerous faculty development programs ranging from new faculty orientations to a Junior Faculty Teaching Fellows program designed to create a community of early-career faculty who learn together how to be more effective and efficient in their teaching (Vanderbilt University, 2019). Vanderbilt's Center for Teaching also provides several teaching guides on topics such as theoretical principles and frameworks of learning and course design, instructional strategies, reflection on and assessment of teaching and learning, challenges and opportunities related to course preparation and classroom management, and understanding the various populations and contexts of higher education.

CAMPUS TRAININGS AND OTHER RESOURCES FOR FACULTY

New Faculty Orientation

Many campuses have a new faculty orientation event at the beginning of each academic year. Although such orientations are often campus-wide events that cover general topics (Moe & Murphy, 2011), you may learn about campus resources that will be useful to you in the future, such as centers for teaching and learning, educational technology departments, and future campus events related to your teaching or research duties.

Preparing Future Faculty

If you are a student in a graduate or professional program, find out if your campus participates in the Preparing Future Faculty program. Launched in 1993 as a partnership between the Council of Graduate Schools and the Association of American Colleges and Universities, Preparing Future Faculty programs originally were designed for students pursuing PhDs in various disciplines who were interested in pursuing faculty roles in the future (Council of Graduate Schools, 2019)). Although initially focused on doctoral students in mathematics, sciences, social sciences, and humanities, hundreds of institutions have implemented similar programs for students across graduate and professional programs. These programs are designed to help students understand the scope of the faculty role and receive mentorship and reflective feedback about their own teaching, research, and service activities.

Faculty Mentoring and Peer Coaching

Some departments have a formal mentoring program established with one or two faculty already designated as mentors for a new faculty member and a set schedule of mentoring activities. For example, the Indiana School of Nursing recently implemented a 3-year mentoring initiative for new faculty to develop their scholarship productivity. Participants attended "five check-in meetings, a summer writing workshop, school and university promotion information sessions, and mentor-protégé meetings" (Shieh & Cullen, 2019, p. 1). Participants were later found to be productive in their scholarship as measured by the number of papers and presentations they had completed during their first few years in their faculty roles. In another study of health professions faculty mentoring, Falzarano and Zipp (2012) found that mentors provided valuable information and support and that mentees appreciated having someone to go to with questions and concerns.

It is much more likely that you will need to seek out these mentoring relationships on your own. If your academic role is more focused on research, find out who has similar research interests. If you were hired primarily for teaching responsibilities, find a few other faculty who can provide guidance about instructional strategies, course planning, and student engagement. It may be helpful to ask if there are other early-career faculty within the department or school. They may be able to offer the most relevant advice to you as a new faculty member because their own struggles with the transition are still fresh in their minds. Seeking mentorship beyond the boundaries of your own department can be very beneficial, but Moe and Murphy (2011) also cautioned the following:

> it is politically astute to listen more and talk less . . . until gaining a bit more familiarity with the environment of the university. It could be devastating to inadvertently insult a potential ally and confidant because one is unfamiliar with the history between departments, people, and issues/policies. (pp. 65)

Professional Association Conferences

Look for opportunities to attend professional association conferences at the state and national levels (Moe & Murphy, 2011). You likely will find workshops, presentations, and posters focused on faculty development specific to your own discipline. Some professional associations have developed entire conferences focused on education within a particular discipline. For example, the American Physical Therapy Association hosts an annual Education Leadership Conference, and the American Occupational Therapy Association hosts an annual Education Summit. Both conferences offer numerous professional development opportunities for faculty in those disciplines.

In addition to the knowledge you will gain from presentations at professional association conferences, you also will have the opportunity to network with faculty in your discipline from other institutions across the state and nation. Take advantage of the time in between sessions to introduce yourself to other attendees. If you find someone with common interests, invite that person to lunch, dinner, or happy hour. Make an effort to keep in touch after the conference to discuss challenges, share resources, bounce ideas off each other, and perhaps pursue educational research together in the future.

RESOURCES SPECIFIC TO YOUR PROFESSION RELATED TO EDUCATION

In addition to attending state and national conferences, find out if your professional association offers any professional development programs for educators. For example, the Academy of Physical Therapy Education offers an annual New Faculty Development Workshop "that facilitates an understanding of the roles and responsibilities of faculty in higher education" (American Physical Therapy Association, 2019, para. 2). The American Occupational Therapy Association offers a four-module *Clinician to Educator Series* (Henderson, 2017) that provides an overview of higher education, professional education, and accreditation standards, learning theories and instructional design strategies, and assessment strategies for teaching and learning relevant for occupational therapy educators.

Your profession may also have a peer-reviewed journal specific to educators in your discipline. For example, *Respiratory Care Education Annual* is a refereed journal "committed to providing a forum for research and theory in respiratory care education," which "showcases scholarly work with the educational community to promote best practices and research in respiratory care education" (American Association for Respiratory Care, 2019, para. 1). Other discipline-specific education journals include *Athletic Training Education Journal*, *Journal of Occupational Therapy Education*, and *Pharmacy Education*, just to name a few.

CONFERENCES FOR NEW FACULTY

Beyond your own discipline's professional association conferences, there are many other faculty development conferences and workshops targeted specifically at health professions educators. For example, the University of Indianapolis hosts the Institute for Emerging Educators in Health Care conference (University of Indianapolis, 2018). Other conferences are open to faculty across higher education, such as the biannual conferences of the New England Faculty Development Consortium (2019). You may have to do a little research to locate conferences in your state or region that are realistic for you to attend in terms of registration and travel costs.

Pursuing an Advanced Degree

Your profession may have specific accreditation standards related to the qualifications of faculty within educational programs. For example, for several years, my profession's accrediting body required at least 50% of full-time faculty teaching in entry-level master's occupational therapy programs to hold a doctoral degree. As my profession moves toward an entry-level clinical doctorate for occupational therapists, all full-time faculty will be required to have a doctorate. This meant that several faculty within my department, including myself, had to pursue an advanced degree over the past few years in order to help our department maintain compliance with accreditation standards. Some elected to pursue a clinical doctorate within our discipline via distance education. I found a part-time PhD program in educational leadership on my own campus that fit well with my work schedule and career goals. Talk with your department chair and colleagues to determine if you will need to pursue an advanced degree in the near future. The following factors should be considered when deciding on the right degree program for you:

- Is obtaining an advanced degree required or simply encouraged?
- Is a particular degree more highly valued by your discipline or institution?
- Are there accreditation implications for your department if you decide not to pursue an advanced degree?
- Do you prefer on-campus or distance education?
- How long will it take you to complete the degree?
- How does required coursework fit in with your work and family obligations?
- How much will it cost, and will your employer provide any tuition assistance?
- Will your employer provide other support while you complete your degree, such as a reduced teaching load?
- Will obtaining an advanced degree have any impact on your salary in the future?

Books and Other Publications

An online search will reveal dozens of books and other resources about college teaching on everything from engaging students to managing large lecture courses to reflective readings on what it means to be a teacher. I try to read at least one new book per year and implement something that I learned from that book into the courses that I teach.

LEARNING ACTIVITIES

1. Explore your campus website for professional development resources related to teaching. Is there a center for teaching? If not, explore the websites for centers for teaching at other institutions. What resources can you locate that may benefit you in the future?

2. Find out if your campus has a faculty mentoring program. Is it formal in nature? Are there specific expectations of mentors and mentees?

3. Go to the website for your national professional association. Are there conferences or other professional development opportunities specific for individuals making a transition into an academic role? What is the cost and time commitment for participating in these opportunities?

4. Identify a list of four or five books related to college teaching that you would like to read over the next several years. How will you prioritize which one to read first?

5. Given the various resources that you have identified for professional development related to your faculty role, create a 5-year professional development plan for yourself. Which conferences will you attend and when? Which books will you read? Which campus workshops will you attend? How will you seek out mentoring?

REFERENCES

American Association for Respiratory Care. (2019). *Respiratory care education annual*. Retrieved from https://www.aarc.org/wp-content/uploads/2019/09/rcea2019.pdf

American Physical Therapy Association. (2019). Faculty development. Retrieved from http://www.apta.org/Educators/Academic/FacultyDevelopment

Council of Graduation Schools. (2019). The Preparing Future Faculty program. Retrieved from https://www.preparing-faculty.org

Falzarano, M., & Zipp, G. P. (2012). Perceptions of mentoring of full-time occupational therapy faculty in the United States. *Occupational Therapy International, 19*(3), 117-126. doi:10.1002/oti.1326

Henderson, W. (2017). *Clinician to educator series set: Modules I, II, III, & IV*. Bethesda, MD: AOTA Press.

Moe, A. M., & Murphy, L. M. (2011). Being a new faculty. In E. Lenning, S. Brightman, & S. Caringella (Eds.), *A guide to surviving a career in academia: Navigating the rites of passage*. New York, NY: Routledge.

New England Faculty Development Consortium. (2019). Upcoming conferences. Retrieved from https://nefdc.org/conferences

Shieh, C., & Cullen, D. (2019). Mentoring nurse faculty: Outcomes of a three-year clinical track faculty initiative. *Journal of Professional Nursing, 35*(3), 162-169.

University of Indianapolis. (2018). Institute for Emerging Educators in Healthcare. Retrieved from https://www.uindy.edu/health-sciences/ieeh/index

University of Missouri Career Center. (2019). Wakonse conference on college teaching. Retrieved from http://wakonse.org

University of Missouri System. (2016). University of Missouri faculty scholars: About the program. Retrieved from https://www.umsystem.edu/ums/aa/faculty/about

Vanderbilt University. (2019). Center for teaching. Retrieved from https://cft.vanderbilt.edu

14

Maintaining Balance in Your Life

"One should be a professor for the love of teaching and research. If one is working too hard to enjoy it then something is wrong" (Project Kaleidoscope, 2009, p. 2).

In addition to my love for teaching others, one of the main reasons I made the transition from clinical practice to academia was to have a better work–life balance. I had been working at an acute care hospital for several years, and all the occupational therapists, physical therapists, and speech-language pathologists in my rehabilitation department were expected to work occasional weekends and holidays. Hospitals do not operate only Monday through Friday from 8:00 a.m. to 5:00 p.m.; patients have needs for medical care, therapy, diagnostic tests, respiratory care, and countless other procedures 365 days per year. At the time I was exploring a transition to academia, my children were in elementary school. Working weekends meant that I missed out on some of their extracurricular activities at least monthly. It also meant that I could not enjoy leisure activities with my husband, who worked Monday through Friday, as often I would have liked. Landing a full-time faculty position at a nearby 4-year university was a dream come true. At the time, I had no idea that many academics find work–life balance elusive.

Scholars have researched and written about the concept of achieving balance between academic work and personal life for years. Not surprisingly, a better work–life balance is correlated with a greater intent to remain in an academic profession (Lindfelt, Gomez, & Barnett, 2018). However, other scholars simply say that work–life balance does not exist.

Gateley, C. A. *Clinical Practice to Academia: A Guide for New and Aspiring Health Professions Faculty* (pp. 199-211). © 2021 Taylor & Francis Group.

You have only one life. Nobody gets a "work life" and a "home life"—don't expect to separate the two. The best you can get is one life that is somewhat balanced, at any given time, between competing needs and desires. (Drexel University, n.d., para. 2)

You'll spot that I haven't mentioned "work–life balance." I don't believe in it. There are only 24 hours in a day, and it's all my life. My work is my life, my home is my life, my family is my life and my addiction to mid-century Belgian ceramics on eBay is also my life. A confluence of luck, good choices, hard work, and support have meant that … it's not terribly stressful to be an academic working mother. (Terras, 2012, para. 12)

Ultimately, you have to decide what "balance" means to you. This chapter explores some of the issues you may encounter as you begin an academic career and provides suggestions for how to minimize feelings of imbalance when work and personal commitments conflict with one another.

DEFINING BALANCE

People define balance in different ways. Balance is not a fixed value; it changes over time, and faculty need to reassess often what is important to them at their particular career and life stages (Project Kaleidoscope, 2009). I certainly have found this true in my own life. When I first started my academic position, I was thrilled to have weekends free to spend more time with family. However, 1 year later, I enrolled in a PhD program and suddenly had many hours of reading and writing to do every week. For the next 5 years as my kids progressed through middle and high school and got more involved in sports and other extracurricular activities, I had to adjust my daily schedule to meet all of my obligations as a spouse, mother, professor, and graduate student. I knew that I did my best learning very early in the morning or very late at night when there were no other distractions, so I set my alarm early to tackle assigned readings or stayed up after the kids went to bed to write a paper.

After I completed my doctorate, my focus again returned to balancing work and family life. "Long academic working hours are legendary. But so are their flexibility" (Terras, 2012, para. 4). Sometimes I left work a little early to travel to a basketball or soccer game, but I often graded quizzes and papers while my husband drove or while I was sitting in the bleachers waiting for a game to begin. I occasionally took entire days off from work to chaperone school field trips or help decorate for prom, knowing that I could spend a few hours in the evening or on the weekend working on a class presentation, developing a new assignment, or responding to work-related emails to make up for missed time at the office. Occasionally, I had to miss one of my kids' events because I had an evening class or campus presentation, but my husband would text me updates that I could check during breaks. One of my favorite places to do brainstorming and preparation for a new course is sitting at a picnic table early in the morning when my husband and I are camping and he is busy fishing in the stream nearby or reading a book. These are just a few examples of how I find balance not by trying to separate my various roles but rather by trying to integrate them.

My sense of balance and strategies to maintain it also changed as my academic career progressed. My university has a promotion process for non–tenure-track faculty with criteria for advancement from, in my particular case, assistant teaching professor to associate teaching professor to teaching professor. In order to achieve promotion at each level, I had to demonstrate excellent teaching and service to my school, campus, and profession. Although research is not an expectation for my particular non–tenure-track position, engagement in any scholarly activity also helped my dossier for promotion. These expectations meant participating in campus recruitment and orientation events, serving on multiple national committees for my professional association, traveling to attend and present at professional conferences, and finding time to write or revise a few textbooks, like the one you are reading now. In order to meet these expectations, I had to reduce some of my other commitments, such as cutting back on the number of times I volunteered for events at my kids' school. More recently, I have encountered some of the challenges of having aging parents and grandparents with health concerns. Accordingly, over the past few years, I declined some professional opportunities that I otherwise would have pursued in order to have more time to attend to their needs.

My story is not unique. I have many roles, each with its own set of expectations. My roles have changed over time, and the expectations of each role have changed over time. Talk to any faculty member, and he or she will have a similar story of competing pressures and ways to seek balance. The remainder of this chapter focuses on advice that other faculty and I have found helpful in our academic roles.

TIPS FOR ACHIEVING AND MAINTAINING BALANCE

Understand the Expectations of Your Academic Position

In retrospect, I had absolutely no idea what I was getting myself into when I applied for a faculty position. I did not know the questions I should have asked during my interview or throughout my first few months in my new position. As it turned out, I still love my role in academia, but much of what I learned through trial and error can be gleaned through interview questions and early conversations with the department chair and other departmental faculty. The following are some examples of questions to ask:

- What classes will I be expected to teach?
- How many classes will I be expected to teach each semester? Does that expectation vary?
- What service responsibilities, such as serving on committees, will I have? Do those expectations change over time?
- What are the expectations for participation in research and other scholarly activities?

- Are there other expectations of this role beyond teaching, service, and scholarship that I should be aware of?
- How do you see this position evolving over time?
- What is a typical work schedule for this position? Does that change during summers and other breaks in the academic calendar?
- What processes are in place for promotion and/or tenure for this type of position? What are the timelines and expectations for promotion?
- How often will I have a performance review, and which areas will be assessed?
- What is the culture of the department, school, and campus surrounding work–life balance?
- What do faculty like best about working here?
- What is most challenging about being a faculty member?
- What surprised you the most about transitioning from clinical practice to academia?
- What kind of orientation will I receive?
- Are there any programs in place to connect me with other new faculty at the department, school, or campus levels?
- What advice would you give to someone like me who is considering transitioning from clinical practice to a faculty position?

Exploring the issues addressed in the previous list of questions before you accept an academic position will give you a better sense of whether that position is a good fit for you and whether you are a good fit for the department's needs.

> We fit in our environment and flourish in our job if it fits with our values and needs and if our abilities match those needed and rewarded in our environment.... We do a great service to our doctoral students and young faculty if we help them examine what type of university they prefer and how they might fit the needs of the position as it fits within their value system. (Hooper & O'Meara, 2009, para. 3)

Set Personal and Professional Goals

Only you can define what work–life balance means to you. Gahrmann (2018) recommended that you should "create harmony in your life—a mixture of work, family and friends. Remember, there is no single formula for balancing work and family. It is a personal decision how one combines spouse, children and career" (para. 11). Much of the literature available on work–life balance for faculty is focused on young females who are balancing family responsibilities with their careers. Hooper and O'Meara (2009) cautioned that discussion about work–life balance should not be limited to young, female faculty. Rather, such discussions should encompass age, gender, sexual orientation, minority status, rank, and career phase. They emphasized that life enjoyment brought about through avocational pursuits also contributes significantly to the work–life balance that faculty experience.

Knowing that you define your own work–life balance, think about where you currently are both personally and professionally, and then set goals for where you would like to be in a few months or a few years. If you are considering a career transition to academia, what aspects of a faculty position would contribute to your personal and professional goals? Do you want more time with family? Do you want more time to pursue leisure activities with friends? Do you want a flexible schedule that allows you to work from home occasionally or to pursue an advanced degree in your discipline? Do you want to start leading a healthier lifestyle through better diet and more exercise? If you are already in academia, what are the competing forces for your time and energy? Are there changes you can make to improve your feeling of balance? What goals do you have for professional advancement? Do you see yourself in an academic leadership position in the future? Do you want to become more involved in your profession at the state or national level?

Regardless of your personal and professional goals, you need to write them down. Individuals who write down their goals are much more likely to accomplish them (Acton, 2017; Pros, 2015). Acton (2017) recommended using the SMART method of goal writing, which stands for the following:

- S–Specific
- M–Measurable
- A–Actionable
- R–Realistic
- T–Timely

Acton also provided the following five tips for improving accountability and the likelihood that you will achieve your goals:

1. Make them visible: It does not help to write down your goals if you never see them. Acton suggested creating an artistic visual representation of your goals. "This activates a different part of your brain, and as it will be wildly different to your working style, will help cement your goals in your mind" (Acton, 2017, para. 2). I am not the least bit artistically inclined and prefer to have a simple handwritten list posted near my desk. You could even set your computer screen saver to show a list of your goals so you are periodically reminded of them.

2. Feel them: Consider writing out a short paragraph about how it would feel to achieve each goal. "Acting like you have already achieved your goal will start to connect the dots between where you are now and the steps you need to take to achieve your goals" (Acton, 2017, para. 3).

3. Understand them: Think about what motivated you to set each goal. Why do you want to achieve it? What will happen if you do not achieve this goal within your desired time frame?

4. Take action: Once you have written your goals, take immediate action, even if it is only a small step toward one of your goals. "Momentum begets momentum, and by kick starting your goal writing process with a tangible action, you will immediately create a sense of progress" (Acton, 2017, para. 5). Review your goals at least monthly to track and celebrate your progress.
5. Share them: Sharing your goals with someone else will help keep you accountable. For personal goals, share them with a family member or trusted friend. For professional goals, share them with a colleague or mentor.

Build a Strong Support System and Use It When Needed

I was extremely lucky to have a supportive spouse during my transition to a faculty position, for my many years in graduate school, and throughout my ongoing academic career. Terras (2012) explained that having a supportive life partner or other family member who can help with chores and childcare is essential to feeling more balanced in your academic position. If you have children, Nagpal (2013) recommended setting up a plan with your partner regarding childcare responsibilities. She and her spouse decided that when one parent was "on duty" for childcare, all responsibilities and decisions fell to that person, and the other parent would not question anything. Additionally, when one parent was "off duty," he or she could schedule that time as needed for work or leisure without guilt. They also made a rule for no work on weekends, except when one of them was required to travel for work. Whenever exceptions to their schedule occurred, such as when one spouse had to care for the kids alone for an entire weekend, that spouse earned a free weekend to be scheduled however he or she wanted or needed to.

Other family and friends can play just as big of a role in helping you with personal commitments (Gahrmann, 2018). Perhaps you have parents or siblings you can lean on occasionally for help with managing hectic schedules that inevitably come with having children. A few of my academic colleagues with young children regularly call on their parents to help with drop-off and pickup from daycare or school. I did not have family who lived nearby when my children were young, but I learned to make friends with the parents of kids who were involved in the same activities as mine. When the occasional crisis situation arose at work and my husband was out of town, I could send a text message to a group of trusted friends to ask if someone could pick up my daughter from school or practice, make sure she got something to eat, and got home safely or remained at a friend's house until I could get there. I would always tell my rescuer, "I may not be able to pay back the favor, but I will try to pay it forward." In addition to helping with personal commitments, if you have had a challenging week at work, an evening out with friends or colleagues may be just the pick-me-up you need to get through the rest of the semester.

If you do not have family or friends that you can rely on for childcare, remember that you have easy access to a bunch of high-achieving, responsible college students. I recommend that you avoid hiring your own current students for babysitting or house-sitting, which could open you up to complaints of favoritism or more serious allegations of impropriety, but I have reached out to former students and students from other health professions programs within our school to have a running list of potential childcare providers when needed. Be sure to read through relevant policies and check with your department chair to make sure you are not violating any campus or department policies for faculty-student contact.

Learn to Say "No"

One of the most important skills in avoiding imbalance in your life is learning to say "no," even to attractive opportunities, if you will find yourself overcommitted by saying "yes" (Gahrmann, 2018; Nagpal, 2013; Project Kaleidoscope, 2009). As a new faculty member, it may be difficult to determine which opportunities you can decline. Committee service will likely be an expectation of your faculty position, but if someone other than your department chair asks you to serve on a committee, task force, or other project, you need to seriously consider whether adding another commitment to your growing list of responsibilities is in your best interest. Is it something you want to do? Will agreeing to this opportunity affect your ability to meet other expectations at work or home? Is this activity something that will look good on your curriculum vitae when you next submit your dossier for promotion?

The longer you are at an institution, the more likely you will be called on for additional service opportunities, particularly if you consistently have agreed to serve in the past. For example, years ago I volunteered to serve on several 1-hour faculty panel discussions with parents of entering freshmen during summer orientation. The student services department of our school of health professions recognized that I enjoyed such events, and soon I was asked to assist with outreach programs to high school students, career fairs, first-year programs for minority students interested in the health professions, and other various campus and community service events. I enjoy representing my profession and interacting with potential students and families, but I have learned to politely decline some opportunities with, "Thank you for thinking of me for this opportunity, but I have a lot of work and personal commitments right now and cannot dedicate the amount of time needed for this additional commitment."

You will also encounter several opportunities for scholarship and service to your profession at the state and national level. For example, a faculty colleague may invite you to participate on a research project with the potential for publication. You may be asked to serve in a leadership position for your state or national professional association or your state licensure board. You may receive invitations to serve as a reviewer for article submissions to a professional journal or proposals to a professional conference. Each one of these opportunities is an excellent way to build your curriculum vitae, but each one will take time away from the primary responsibilities of your faculty position and other life roles. One academic cautioned, "When you are on your death bed, is it more likely that you will wish you had written a few more papers or had spent more time with your kids?" (Project Kaleidoscope, 2009, p. 1).

Nagpal (2013) provided several suggestions for setting limits on work. First, she travels for work no more than five times per year, meaning that she must consider carefully which professional conferences are most important for her to attend. She has a quota for nonteaching, nonresearch items. For example, she sets limits on the number of papers she will review, the number of events with which she will assist, and the number of panels on which she will serve. It "makes you think a lot before you say 'yes'" (Nagpal, 2013, p. 6). She also has a weekly hard vs. fun quota: "If I can do one hard thing and one fun thing per week, then I declare victory" (Nagpal, 2013, p. 6).

One limit that I set to help maintain balance in my life was the decision to not have my work email set up on my cell phone. On any given day, I receive 20 to 50 emails to my work email address. I have colleagues who report daily numbers over 100. Many of those emails come outside of the hours when I am at my office, and many of them are emails that do not require my attention or a response, such as school- or campus-wide daily or weekly announcements. If I checked my phone every time a work email arrived in my inbox, it would add up to dozens of interruptions during my personal time with friends and family. My department chair and colleagues all know my decision, and they know they can text me anytime if there is something that requires my immediate attention. My students also know my policy, and I inform them on the first day of the semester that I will respond to emails Monday through Friday 7:30 a.m. to 4:00 p.m.; I make occasional exceptions to that policy when there is an upcoming exam and I know that students may have more questions than usual, but in those instances, I explain to students that I will check and respond to emails once per evening. Obviously, you need to verify with your department chair what the expectations are for your particular position, but this decision definitely had a positive effect on my personal sense of work–life balance.

You will need to determine what your limits are. Gahrmann (2018) emphasized the importance of living by your own standards, rather than someone else's, and establishing boundaries. "Boundaries are an imaginary line of protection that you draw around yourself. They are about protecting you from other people's actions" (Gahrmann, 2018, para. 4). In many cases, the quality of your work is way more important than the quantity of your work. "Whatever you are doing—in research or in education—do it extraordinarily well. Make it high quality. Make sure what you do is documented to make you visible as a valuable faculty member" (Project Kaleidoscope, 2009, p. 1).

Avoid Guilt

Closely related to saying "no" to help maintain work–life balance is avoiding guilt for the decisions you make. Gahrmann (2018) explained that "guilt is one of the greatest wastes of emotional energy" (para. 3). It is okay to say no to a professional opportunity. It is okay to miss a few of your kids' extracurricular activities. It is okay to miss work when a family member is sick and needs you to be at home. Terras (2012) dispelled what she called the *Superwoman fallacy* for women in academia, explaining that she experiences no guilt in paying for extra help, such as a weekly house cleaner, or taking shortcuts when possible. She bragged that she has not ironed a single article of clothing since 2003, and no one has noticed.

You cannot be all things to all people at all times. Occasionally, you will not meet the expectations that others have set for you or that you have set for yourself. Life does go on. As I type this sentence, I am more than 1 year beyond the deadline I originally set with the publisher for this manuscript; yet, it will still get published. The original deadline, and a few subsequent deadlines, fell at a time when I was incredibly busy preparing my department for reaccreditation and compiling my dossier for promotion, my youngest daughter was in the middle of deciding which out-of-state college she would attend, my oldest daughter was exploring options for graduate school, a close family member had recently passed away and I was dealing with her estate, my parents were faced with some serious health issues that resulted in the decision for my husband and I to sell our home and move into a new home with them, and my husband was diagnosed with stage IV cancer and undergoing chemotherapy treatments. With all of those work and family responsibilities pulling me in different directions, I was not able to dedicate the time I needed to work on this book, and I lost my "writing mojo" for several months. Thankfully, I had an understanding editor and publisher who assured me that I should not feel guilty about tending to other important responsibilities in my life. Whenever you find yourself overwhelmed with responsibilities, take a step back, prioritize, and initiate conversations with the appropriate people if you need to make some adjustments to your commitments.

Use Technology to Make Your Life Easier

Terras (2012) emphasized that you should "make technology your friend" (para. 8). Smartphones are commonplace for most working adults, but if you are transitioning from clinical practice to academia, you may not be used to using an electronic calendar to manage your daily schedule. Or perhaps you had a shared calendar with a spouse or partner, but you have never experienced having dozens of people with access to your daily calendar. Whatever email and calendar system your institution uses, learn how to use it. In addition to organizing daily and weekly schedules, you may need to develop a running to-do list of future commitments to keep track of priorities (Gahrmann, 2018).

Technology can be used to maintain work–life balance in other ways beyond daily schedules and to-do lists (Terras, 2012). You can use a laptop, tablet, or cell phone to respond to emails and complete other work-related tasks when you are waiting at a doctor's office or sitting on an airplane. You can video chat with your family and friends when you are working late at the office or out of town for work.

Some people prefer low-tech strategies to manage personal and work commitments. Several of my departmental colleagues have to-do lists and schedules ranging from a simple list on a small wipe-off board near the computer to elaborate grids on magnetic whiteboards to keep track of upcoming deadlines for grants, article submissions, committee projects, and teaching responsibilities. Although I rely heavily on my electronic calendar for work, my family and I still use a central paper calendar to remember who is doing what on any given day. A faculty friend of mine with five young children has an impressive color-coded calendar that she and her spouse use to coordinate work and family events. Do what works best for you!

Schedule Time for Whatever You Need to Accomplish

When I first started in my faculty position, the only things I put on my electronic calendar were classes and meetings, which made it look like I had 20 to 25 hours of "free time" each week. I have since learned the importance of scheduling time for everything I need to accomplish, not just the things that require my attendance. If I need to create an assignment for a class, I block out time on my calendar. If I need to grade exams or assignments, I block out time on my calendar.

If research and publication are important for your role, block out time on your calendar for those activities. "Just as teaching commitments get scheduled and have to be met, so too should writing, reading, and researching be scheduled, with those commitments taking priority over any unscheduled activities" (Project Kaleidoscope, 2009, p. 2). If you agree to write a letter of recommendation for a student or colleague, block out time for that. If you need to review a submission to an academic journal or professional conference, block out time for that. Having a visual reminder of what you need to accomplish in a given day, week, or month makes it much easier to judge when you may need to work late, when you need to say "no" to an opportunity, or when you can take a day off to spend with family.

When my kids were involved in sports and other school activities, I put every single kid event on my electronic calendar as soon as their schedules were available. I knew that I likely would not make it to every event, but having that visual reminder on my calendar weeks or months in advance made it easier for me to schedule committee meetings and other work responsibilities at times that would not impact my ability to attend events that were important to my family. In addition to scheduling family commitment, be sure to schedule time for yourself.

> Being a good parent, partner, and professional means being good to yourself first.... Find ways to relax, relieve tension, and minimize stress. Taking some time off for yourself will not only benefit you, but it will benefit your work and family tremendously as well! (Gahrmann, 2018, para. 6)

Use Work Travel Time Effectively

Your faculty position may include the opportunity, or even the expectation, for attendance and presentation at professional conferences. Professional conferences provide a great opportunity for networking with members from your discipline and related disciplines from across the state or country (Jacques, 2013). They also give you the chance to get away from the stress of everyday work and enjoy time with colleagues or time for yourself (American Nurses Association, 2015). However, attending conferences takes away time from both your family and your other work responsibilities. Terras (2012) recommended taking some kind of work along with you when you travel because time alone in a hotel room is a great opportunity to work without the usual distractions encountered at the office. I almost always travel with some kind of work. I can grade papers sitting on a plane or at the airport. I can work on a writing project for a few hours in the evening after attending conference events, doing a little sightseeing in whichever city I am in, and going to happy hour or dinner with new acquaintances or longtime friends.

Always Have a Backup Plan for Your Students

No matter how well prepared you are for teaching a course, chances are something will happen during the semester that changes your planned schedule. You may have a funeral to attend or a family situation that requires an unexpected day or two off from work. I live in the Midwest where winter weather occasionally wreaks havoc and results in my university closing for a day or two. I have colleagues who live in hurricane-prone areas where classes have been canceled for a week or more in the middle of a semester. When an entire institution closes for several days, administration may institute a plan for making up missed time; however, it is always good practice to have a backup plan in place, particularly when you are faced with meeting accreditation requirements for addressing particular subject matter in your course. San Jose State University Center for Faculty Development (2017) recommends the following:

> Have some key class activities that are relevant to your learning objectives to the class but can be worked on without you prepared at the beginning of the semester. Some examples might be watching a relevant video or reading through and answering discussion questions on some related articles. These can be placed into the class period at the last minute if you have an unexpected family commitment. (para. 4)

Create a Feel-Good Folder

Nagpal (2013) recommended creating a "feel-good folder" to help maintain work–life balance. Nagpal had an email folder where she saved emails that made her happy, such as encouraging emails from students and colleagues or emails about accepted awards. Although I had not thought about naming it until I encountered Nagpal's blog post, I have kept a similar feel-good folder over the years. I save all the thank you notes and various cards I receive from students, friends, and faculty. It is not unusual for a student to give you a thank you card for writing them a letter of recommendation. The ones that always surprise me are the thoughtful cards and emails from students as they are leaving our program thanking me for my teaching, advising, and compassion. Occasionally, recent graduates send an email or card thanking me for teaching them something that they found relevant in their first job. These small gestures always serve to remind me why I love my job in academia.

Seek Out Work in Academic Settings That Promote Work–Life Balance and Family-Friendly Policies

Many higher education institutions have recognized the importance of establishing family-friendly policies to recruit and retain faculty and staff. As you search for academic positions, explore campus websites to see if the institution has any policies in place to address work–life balance. For example, the University of Illinois Office of the Provost (2018) has an entire website dedicated to "Work-Life Balance and Family Friendly Programs," such as a childcare resource service, a modified duties policy that allows faculty additional time off after birth or adoption of a child, and a variety of wellness services for faculty and family members.

San Jose State University's Center for Faculty Development (2017) also has a web page of resources aimed at helping faculty achieve a good sense of work–life balance. The website of Delaware Technical Community College (2018) defines work–life balance as "the ideal arrangement of an individual's employment schedule and private time to facilitate health and personal satisfaction without negatively affecting productivity, professional success, or student success" (para. 1) and has established a set of guidelines for department chairs and faculty to follow as they collaborate to determine work expectations. The University of Pennsylvania Office of the Provost (2018) has a snow day childcare option for faculty and staff when the university is open but public schools are closed. The same institution also has a subsidy program to help offset the cost of childcare or elder care so employees can meet work responsibilities. These are just a few examples of the many policies and practices that higher education institutions have put into place to address the growing demand from employees and potential employees for work–life balance.

LEARNING ACTIVITIES

1. Search the website of the institution where you currently hold an academic position or hope to hold an academic position. Do you find any evidence of family-friendly policies such as those described in this chapter to help faculty achieve work–life balance?

2. If possible, interview a faculty member and ask about that individual's perception of work–life balance in an academic position.

3. Think about your personal and professional goals for the next 5 years. Write down at least two or three goals for each category using the SMART method described in this chapter. Who will you share these goals with?

4. Think about the balance, or lack thereof, you feel in your own life right now. Write down a list of the roles you have. Which roles get most of your time and attention? Are you happy with that? What changes would you like to see? How can you accomplish those goals?

5. Identify one thing you can do in the immediate future (within the next week) that will give you a better sense of work–life balance. Can you go out on a date with your spouse or significant other? Can you go to lunch or a movie with a friend? Can you let your kids choose a fun activity for an upcoming weekend? Can you take a bath and read a book tonight?

REFERENCES

Acton, A. (2017, November 3). How to set goals (and why you should write them down). *Forbes.* Retrieved from https://www.forbes.com/sites/annabelacton/2017/11/03/how-to-set-goals-and-why-you-should-do-it

American Nurses Association. (2015). Professional networking for nurses. Retrieved from https://www.nursingworld.org/resources/individual/networking

Delaware Technical Community College. (2018). Work life balance. Retrieved from https://www.dtcc.edu/about/employment/work-life-balance

Drexel University. (n.d.). Finding your own work-life fit. Retrieved from https://drexel.edu/facultyaffairs/work-life-fit/finding-your-own-work-life-balance/

Gahrmann, N. A. (2018). The top 10 tips for balancing work and family life. MomMD. Retrieved from https://www.mommd.com/10waysbalancework.shtml

Hooper, C. R., & O'Meara, K. (2009). *Balancing faculty careers and work lives.* American Speech-Language-Hearing Association. Retrieved from https://www.asha.org/ArticlesBalancing-Faculty-Careers-and-Work-Lives/

Jacques, S. (2013, March 27). Networking strategies for medical professionals. Physicians Practice. Retrieved from http://www.physicianspractice.com/pearls/networking-strategies-medical-professionals

Lindfelt, T., Gomez, A., & Barnett, M. J. (2018). The impact of work-life balance on intention to stay in academia: Results from a national survey of pharmacy faculty. *Research in Social and Administrative Pharmacy, 14*(4), 387-390. doi:10.1016/j.sapharm.2017.04.008

Nagpal, R. (2013, July 21). The awesomest 7-year postdoc or: How I learned to stop worrying and love the tenure-track life. *Scientific American.* Retrieved from https://blogs.scientificamerican.com/guest-blog/the-awesomest-7-year-postdoc-or-how-i-learned-to-stop-worrying-and-love-the-tenure-track-faculty-life

Project Kaleidoscope. (2009). Balancing your career & personal life. Swarthmore. Retrieved from https://www.swarthmore.edu/sites/default/files/assets/documents/faculty-diversity-excellence/BalancingCareer.pdf

Pros, D. (2015, June 30). 5 reasons why writing down goals increases the odds of achieving them. Elite Daily. Retrieved from https://www.elitedaily.com/money/writing-down-your-goals/1068863

San Jose State University Center for Faculty Development. (2017). Work life balance resources. http://www.sjsu.edu/cfd/career-planning/work-life-balance/family-matters/WLBworklifebalance/index.html

Terras, M. (2012). The Superwoman fallacy: What it really takes to be an academic and parent. *The Guardian.* Retrieved from https://www.theguardian.com/higher-education-network/blog/2012/aug/17/academic-careers-work-life-balance

University of Illinois Office of the Provost. (2018). Work-life balance and family-friendly programs. https://provost.illinois.edu/faculty-affairs/work-life-balance/#sthash.piOoeEEt.dpbs

University of Pennsylvania Office of the Provost. (2018). Work-life balance. Retrieved from https://provost.upenn.edu/faculty/current/work-life-balance

Index

Printed in the United States
by Baker & Taylor Publisher Services